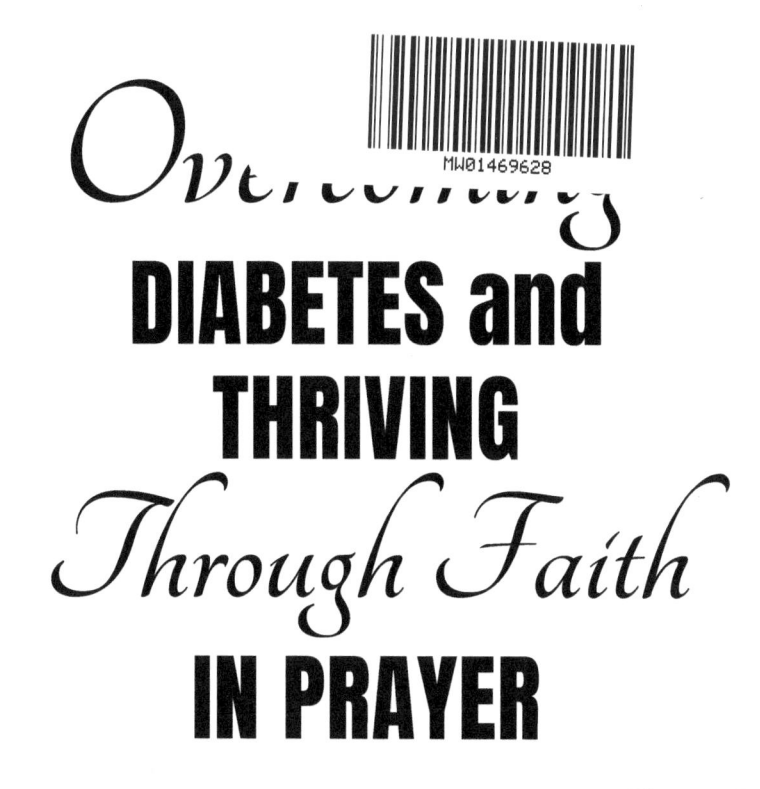

Overcoming DIABETES and THRIVING Through Faith IN PRAYER

God Bless Your Family

Dwight Treadwell

TRUE STORY *by Dwight Treadwell*
THE ENIGMA

TRILOGY
PROFESSIONAL PUBLISHING MEETS POWERFUL PROMOTION

A wholly owned subsidiary of TBN

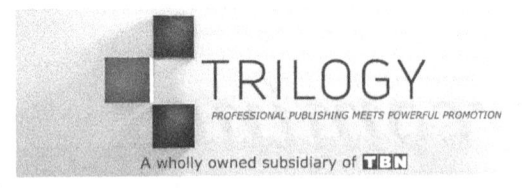

No part of this publication may be reproduced, stored in a retrieval system, or transmitted in any way nor by any means, electronically, mechanically, photocopied, recorded, or otherwise, without the prior permission of the Authors as provided by the USA copyright law.

Trilogy Christian Publishers

A Wholly Owned Subsidiary of Trinity Broadcasting Network

2442 Michelle Drive | Tustin, CA 92780

Copyright © 2025 by Dwight Treadwell

All Scripture quotations, unless otherwise noted, are taken from The Holy Bible, King James Version. Cambridge Edition: 1769.

Scripture quotations marked TLB are taken from The Living Bible copyright © 1971. Used by permission of Tyndale House Publishers, a Division of Tyndale House Ministries, Carol Stream, Illinois 60188. All rights reserved.

All rights reserved, including the right to reproduce this book or portions thereof in any form whatsoever.

For information, address Trilogy Christian Publishing

Rights Department, 2442 Michelle Drive, Tustin, CA 92780.

Trilogy Christian Publishing/ TBN and colophon are trademarks of Trinity Broadcasting Network.

For information about special discounts for bulk purchases, please contact Trilogy Christian Publishing.

Trilogy Disclaimer: The views and content expressed in this book are those of the author and may not necessarily reflect the views and doctrine of Trilogy Christian Publishing or the Trinity Broadcasting Network.

10 9 8 7 6 5 4 3 2 1

Library of Congress Cataloging-in-Publication Data is available.

ISBN 979-8-89597-384-4 | ISBN 979-8-89597-385-1 (ebook)

Dedication

This book is dedicated to my parents and is in memory of my father, the late Robert Lane Treadwell, Sr. (1933–2011). Dad was affectionately called Rob by his parents, siblings, and a host of cousins. He was born in the heart of the bustling steel mill industry of Birmingham, Alabama, on August 22, 1933. Dad was from a traditional two-parent household, including four sisters and one brother. Also, in the 1930s–40s, most of his relatives lived in the same neighborhood, as close as right next door. My father and mother moved our family to Detroit, Michigan, in the early 1950s for better-paying jobs in the emerging automobile industry. Dad was fortunate to get hired by the General Motors Company. He garnered respect for being a dependable, courteous, and dedicated employee. He was employed with General Motors for over thirty years—until they semi-forced him into retirement only because of health issues. It is ironic that Dad left the city (Birmingham) that produced steel to wind up in the city (Detroit) that used steel to produce automobiles.

My parents were known for their dedication to God and family, and for their prosperous lifestyles.

Dad was kind and incredibly generous with his time

and resources. He was an avid bowler, and as his skills increased, he and his four-person team were a unit to be reckoned with; they traveled throughout the country, participating in tournaments.

Table of Contents

Preamble 9

Introduction. 13

First Quarter 15

The Early Days Of "Carefree Living" 19

Mid-Adolescence Competitive Years 21

Confusion About The Term "Sugar". 25

Activity In Sports 29

Diabetes Acknowledgment 33

Religion. 35

Second Quarter 43

The Verdict Was Cast 45

Why Is Forty-Five The Magic Age For Diabetes? 49

What Are The Early Symptoms Of Diabetes? 51

Climbing Up The Rough Side Of The Mountain
  To Full Recovery. 53

Lifelong Hospital Avoidance 57

Work Environment—Work Ethic 59

How Can You Measure Pain?. 63

Hospital Vampires. 67

Common Cliques 69

Halftime 73

You Do Not Need Medical Training To Be An
  At Home Caregiver. 79

My Caregiver's Point Of View. 81

What Happens When Your Caregiver Gets Sick?. 89

The Caregiver, Historical Account Of "The Sugar"
  Making A House Call 91

Traveling Around The U.S. 95

How Important Is The Support Of Your Spouse/The
  Caregiver. 97

The Spouse-Partner Caregiver 99

Cliques 101

The Second Half 105

Looking Forward To Your Future 109

Verification Of Information..................... 111

Post-Surgery Anecdotal Memories 113

The Ironic Joy Of Thriving Through Devastation ... 121

Overtime 125

Post Amputation Issues........................ 129

Prosthetic Leg Fitting Procedures................ 131

Pre-And Post Surgery Footwear Adjustments 133

Pre-Surgery Procedures........................ 135

Post-Amputation Surgery Food Allergies.......... 139

Covid Infection Avoidance 141

Benefits Of Being Designated As Disabled 143

Contributors 145

Endocrinology 147

Dental Hygiene 149

Diabetic Vision And Eye Care 151

Anesthesiology 153

Home Health Care Perspective 157

Pictorial Journey 163

Testimonials 167

Preamble

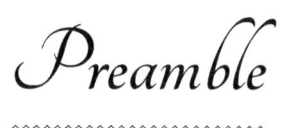

Hello friends, family, and sports fans. The basic construction and design of this book is akin to athletic games, even though the battle against the Sugar is a life-and-death struggle. Yet it has similarities to a sporting contest—all sporting contestants, whether it is football, baseball, basketball, volleyball, or golf for both male and female contestants. Mankind's nature is to fight for dominance. Therefore, you will have winners and losers in these testosterone-fueled contests. All sporting contests will have a beginning and an unknown ending, so it is as we begin to delve into the battle against the Sugar.

The battle started slowly and quietly; it intensified like a football game over time. I will introduce five giants in the soul-saving, encouraging, and inspirational preaching profession that helped me along my journey in the battle versus the Sugar. First is my home church, Pastor Frank Ray, Sr., aka the head coach of the Spirituality Soul Saving Team, aka "the walking Bible," Senior Pastor at New Salem Baptist Church, Memphis, Tennessee. Coach Ray will provide the team with spiritual encouragement and motivation for pressing forward to overcome the sugar "because we are more than conquerors."

Secondly, I would like to introduce the offensive coordinator against the sugar, Bishop Kevin Treadwell, Sr. from Leesburg, Virginia. Bishop Treadwell will stress unto us the power of consistent prayer during troubling times. Thirdly, I would like to introduce my defensive coordinator, Pastor Albert Bry, Jr., Senior Pastor at Second Avenue Baptist Church, Birmingham, Alabama. Yes, he is my first cousin who will be standing in the gap, telling the defensive team about spiritual preparedness for enduring times. This means if diabetes runs in your family, like it does in mine, then you do not need to play around with the Sugar. It is headed your way eventually. So, get prepared now before the Sugar heads your way. Fourthly, our team member Pastor Martin Treadwell will provide for us Sugar sufferers a motivational dissertation at halftime of this battle against the Sugar, realizing that the score is forty to zero in the Sugar's favor, but we are down but NOT out! The battle is not yours but the Lord's. Pastor Martin Treadwell will unearth from his wealth of firsthand knowledge about modern-day miracles, meaning there is yet light at the end of the tunnel for us diabetics. Victory is in our sights.

Sometimes a sporting contest is tied on the scoreboard. Yes, like in all sporting contests, it is also true in this battle against the Sugar! The scoreboard may read that the struggle has come down to an unbreakable tie. The rules state that when the time clock runs out without a clear winner, there must be an overtime period. Therefore, I would like to introduce Bishop Victor Sharpe, Senior Pastor at St. John the Great Baptist Church, Detroit, Michigan. Bishop Sharpe will skillfully guide us through this period. Yes, overtime for diabetes can be defined as "Life or Death hanging in the balance of time."

Therefore, put on your seat belts, buckle up your chin straps, and reach way down in the bucket of faith for intestinal fortitude to press on when the clock of life runs out on you!

Put your seat belts on and enjoy this literary work.

Introduction

Hello, friends and consumers of intellectual information about overcoming illnesses, disorders, catastrophic accidents, and inherited blood defects. It is a philosophical statement that has proven true over the centuries: We all suffer the same illness—it is called the Human Condition. "The Human Condition" is an unavoidable malady. It is not contagious, but all share it! Therefore, illnesses, whatever they are … heart attacks, strokes, cancer, blood diseases, diabetes, lupus, etc., are only the results of living this life. The ultimate Designer of our bodies has time-stamped how long we shall exist in the world! Yes, living a good, clean life helps extend the time clock; medication, exercise, proper diet, etc., are good habits to follow. This book is designed and written to tell you about my journey through the active life of a healthy person—to suffering one of the most devastating effects of diabetes: the amputation of my foot and, eventually, my left leg below the knee. Be inspired through this true story about overcoming and then thriving post-surgery in an area that is usually defined as a death sentence!

Throughout this book, I will refer to diabetes as "the Sugar," the term used to soften the emotional effects of the illness! Then, in chronological order, I will explain how I overcame it and am now thriving in life again. Yes, I am thriving; most of my physical abilities have returned, and I can again stand in the "Winner's Circle" in sports and life. I am an "ENIGMA," also known as an "Ultimate Overcomer." The following pages hopefully will inspire others and encourage them to understand that there is life after a tragedy, and you can be an overcomer!

First Quarter

Dr. Frank E. Ray, Sr.
Head Coach of the Soul Saving and
Inspirational Team
"The Walking Bible"
Memphis, TN

All games have a beginning. Usually, these contests start out slowly, with each contestant jabbing lightly, trying to feel the other contestant out. The battle against sugar truly had little impact on my intellectual acknowledgment of the disease. Also, it was like a young athlete playing in his or her first T-ball or soccer game. After the game, sugary treats were encouraged by the parents of the team.

We Are More Than Conquerors Through The Power Of Prayer

The power of prayer and its specific role of prayer is not just an act of communication; it is an invitation for God's presence to transform situations. It opens the door for divine intervention, allowing God's purpose to unfold through those who pray.

It reflects the importance of invoking God's hand to prepare the hearts and minds of believers to invite the divine into their hearts to seek guidance, wisdom, and strength.

The book of Job is a notable example of being more than a conqueror through the power of prayer, overcoming obstacles. Through Job's confession and repentance, the Lord accepted his prayer.

In Job 42:10, the LORD turned the captivity of Job, when he prayed for his friends giving him twice as much as he had before. Here are six (6) key things that blessed Job's life for 140 more years after he prayed:

1. Fortune—In Job 42:10b, Job received from God twice as much as he had before his trial, which were gifts of friendship and courtesy. Philippians 3:10 says, "That I may know him, and the power of his resurrection, and the fellowship of his sufferings, being made conformable unto his death."

2. Fellowship—Job 42:11 is a transformation of Job's circumstances, as he experienced divine favor again. It is a testament to the complex interplay of suffering, faith, and divine purpose.

3. Friendliness—Job 42:11b, "And they bemoaned

him, and comforted him over all the evil that the LORD had brought upon him: every man also gave him a piece of money, and every one an earring of gold." After Job's trials, his family and friends who had previously distanced themselves came back to show support and solidarity. This signified a restoration of relationships and a return to community following his period of hardship. It taught Job that the journey through suffering can lead to a richer, more profound knowledge of God.

4. Flocks and Food—Job 42:12, "So the Lord blessed the latter end of Job more than his beginning: for he had fourteen thousand sheep, and six thousand camels, and a thousand yoke of oxen, and a thousand she asses." God blessed Job with more at the end of his life than at the beginning.

5. Fair Daughters and Sons—Job 42:13–15, He also had seven sons and three daughters. God gave Job ten more kids, which included seven sons and three beautiful daughters. James 4:14 says, "Whereas ye know not what shall be on the morrow. For what is your life? It is even a vapour, that appeareth for a little time, and then vanisheth away."

6. Fantastic Health and a Full Life—Job 42:16–17 tells us, "After this Job lived one hundred and forty years, and saw his children and grandchildren *for* four generations. So Job died, old and full of days."

Throughout all of his trials, Job retained his integrity and his trust in God even when it was suggested that he "curse God and die" (Job 2:9). Because all of us may feel like Job at one time or another, this book offers a poignant analysis of some of life's most difficult questions.

In a time of trial, God wants us to stick with Him and not give up. God's comforting presence and restoring mercies will eventually come.

Whether in moments of joy, times of need, or in the quiet of a daily routine, prayer is a powerful tool for Christians to deepen their faith, find comfort and guidance, and connect with God. May you continue your individual and communal journeys of faith, letting the profound practice of prayer transform your lives and the lives of others—be blessed.

Dr. Frank E. Ray Sr.

New Salem Baptist Church, Memphis, Tennessee

The Early Days Of "Carefree Living"

I spent my elementary school days as a child playing kickball on the playgrounds. We walked to and from school every day. There was no city or county bus service, not even in inner-city Detroit.

My brothers and friends played softball across the street from our house on Bangor Street in very inner-city Detroit on the vacant lots where two houses used to stand.

All the boys who lived on our street raced up and down the street to crown the speed king of the block. Times were good back then. Each party would have to wrestle with the other to settle the difference when a disagreement occurred. Even the thought of a fistfight was uncommon in the late sixties and early seventies.

When school was released for summer breaks, kids my age and I joined/signed up for summer camp, which was extremely enjoyable. Summer camp meant riding a bus out to River Rouge Park in Detroit, swimming five days a week, and, of course, having swimming contests and diving off the three-tier high diving platform; during the diving contest, I was never great at diving! I always wound up doing belly flops—which was painful. Other great benefits of summer camp were free lunch and afternoon snacks, but most kids my age did not have money for soda machines. So, it was cold water, milk, or box juices for refreshments. The most significant benefit of summer camp was looking at and flirting with the pretty girls in swimsuits!

As the summer break ended, I was ready to go to the multiple secondary and high school levels. The final part of summer recess was the annual family reunion, usually held in Birmingham, Alabama. Even though it was all family, it was ultra-competitive, but for fun, family members on different teams were determined to win. Truly sentimental awards only, not expensive, not recordable in the annals of family history! It was an inter-family gene thing. Which family tree branch had the best gene pool and produced winners?

Mid-Adolescence Competitive Years

Over the years, a young person, male or female, endures body changes and growth spurts of the hair, feet, nose, ears, legs, hands, etc. This age brings about separation and competitive desires and advanced physical abilities among friends and relatives. The ages sixteen and above is when natural hormones engorge the bloodstream and competition for the attention of your peers and of a different sex becomes fierce. Therefore, a youngster, whether male or female, who would or could only run a mile just for fun, at this age, for example, would run 2–3 miles just to see the competition collapse from exhaustion, just to prove who was the alpha male or female of our group!

Right up until my senior year of high school, I was little more than a teetotaler. I barely even drank or consumed half a can of beer. By becoming famous and cool, and one of the in crowd among my peers, I tried to appear mature and worldly. So, I indulged in light drinking of alcohol and light beer. I even tried a little weed. I never cared for smoking anyway.

I knew that college was in my near future, so I wanted to keep a healthy, clean internal system. I dabbled with sex just a tiny bit! I knew that I did not want any babies holding me back from pursuing my college future!

Like many aspiring young athletes, sports drinks were a staple of our rehydration regime. Sports drinks in the 1960s and 70s were loaded with sugar. Back then, the commonly accepted routine was that sugar was good for the body.

I remember at another family reunion gathering when the elder aunts, uncles, and cousins would be in the family room talking about issues of life and how everyone's health was throughout the family, they would quickly usher the children out of the room, saying, "You all need to leave now because grown folk are talking." But we kids were clever, as all kids think they are. We listened at the outer door while grown folks were talking about who had the Sugar. Our eyes popped wide open, thinking, the Sugar?

We would search every room in the house looking for the hidden sugar, whether it was cookies, candy, pies, cakes, ice cream, or sodas. We were determined to find the Sugar.

Because at our age, we enjoyed sugar holidays like

Halloween, Christmas, Easter, July 4, and Thanksgiving. We enjoyed sugar at birthday parties, weddings, and special events as well.

We honestly thought that our parents would not lie about Big Daddy having the Sugar. Therefore, the Sugar is somewhere in the house or in his car, or even hidden in the garage. As devious little rascals, we found all the hidden Christmas gifts, birthday gifts, and the stuff that parents hide that we were not supposed to find. But at last, we had to face defeat and openly admit that we could not find the Sugar that everyone was saying that Big Daddy and others had. For kids our age, it was a crushing defeat. We must openly admit to our peers and other cousins that we kool kids could not find the Sugar, that all the adults were whispering about.

Then, years later, I realized that the Sugar was not a gift or treat. Because it was, and still is, Sugar Diabetes. Whether whispered or spoken aloud.

Confusion About The Term "Sugar"

For several years hanging around my family members at home and traveling with my family, I would hear adults whisper the word "SUGAR." They would say, "Uncle or Cousin got a touch of the Sugar." I would go outside or to my room and think, "You can buy sugar down at the corner grocery store for ten cents a bag!" I wondered, was someone secretly smuggling sugar from other states?

Secondly, more seasoned mothers would tell younger women that in order to help their baby suck milk from their breast, Granny said to sprinkle a little sugar on the nipples—thus came the term "Sugar Tits."

I was a curious teenager, so I tried a lot of homemade cooking recipes. I even signed up for home economics in high school, just to experiment with food. Of course, my favorite dishes were desserts. Even when cooking vegetables, I would add a little teaspoon of sugar to green beans, asparagus, black-eyed peas, carrots, squash, okra—you name it, I added a touch of sugar. So, you see my confusion when people would say, "He got a Touch of the Sugar."

Thirdly, when I really got interested in girls, I became keenly aware of pretty women! The way they wore their clothes and shoes. The way they walked. The way they smelled. So, I considered myself an expert connoisseur of women, and I was always trying to get a little sugar, aka a kiss! But again, I was befuddled. My peers would say to me, "You better watch out—the girl that you are smiling at has a touch of Sugar." So, I had to ask, what does "a touch of the Sugar" really mean?

It was finally explained to me that Sugar, or the touch of Sugar has several meanings.

Example:

A) Family member or friend with a touch of the Sugar, when whispered, means illness!

B) Adding sugar to body parts, male or female sexual parts means stimulation, or in the case of babies or young children eating distasteful foods, sugar means encouragement psychologically.

C) For males and females, having a touch of the Sugar means feminine behavior for males or masculine for females.

Finally, no one ever came out and explained that this common term, the Sugar, for most people, means diabetes, whether spoken aloud or whispered!

Humorously, people would whisper, "He has the Sugar," then scream, "Oh no, not the Sugar!" like Red Fox would say, "It's the Big one!"

Activity In Sports

Yes, by all accounts, I was known by friends and foes as an overly active sports fanatic! I participated in several sports teams for my high school—Detroit Western International High School. In 1972 I was selected as captain of our basketball team, captain of our football team, and also as one of the leaders of our track team. I genuinely enjoyed swimming but did not have a traditional stroke in any of the organized swimming disciplines.

After graduating from high school, which is also known as secondary school, I enrolled at Knoxville College, Knoxville, Tennessee, in the fall of 1973. Even as a first-year player on the football team, I exhibited leadership qualities. I became captain of our college football team as a sophomore and one of the on-campus leaders in my senior year. I was voted most likely to succeed and most athletic in campus superlatives in 1977.

Yes, I also developed what was called a sweet tooth! I was young and extremely active in sports! I never gave the "Sugar Montage" a second thought. Having the Sugar was the old people's problem. I was ignorant of the effects of diabetes. I did not know how to catch it or how to get it. I assumed it was something similar to catching a cold or something. I surely did not think that a twenty-something-year-old could contract the dreaded whispered illness called the Sugar.

For the next twenty-five years of my life, I continued to favor desserts and continued to run, work out, and participate in sports. Really, I felt fine! But just like a well-tuned clock, when I turned forty-five years old, something changed! I was extremely thirsty—a lot more than normal, so I cut down on my consumption of beer. I was only drinking water and a soda every now and then! But I found myself going to the restroom, urinating a lot more than I was consuming liquids. I was losing 8–10 pounds a week through peeing. Finally, I went to my doctor, and I was diagnosed with type 2 diabetes, which is when the pancreas makes less insulin than it used to, and your body becomes resistant to insulin.

I was first recommended for pills and diet change, and more exercise! The doctor said to come back in six months, and if I had improved, he would consider taking me off the pills. I worked out like an Olympian, ate extremely well, lost a few more pounds, then went back to my doctor.

As stated in the previous chapter, sugar was a necessary ingredient for rehydration. Sugar is not listed as a hallucinogenic drug, such as weed, cocaine, LSD, ecstasy, and others. But sugar gives us the calming inner effect of satisfaction or mental fullness. Yes, most Class 1 drugs are highly addictive and will need specialized withdrawal treatments by professionals. "The Sugar," although not a Class 1 or Class 2 addictive drug, is very addictive to most. Breaking free from the grips of the Sugar is as hard as breaking free from strong drugs, alcohol, or even smoking. Sugar is legally encouraged and supported by all facets of human consumption. There are no laws currently against sugar.

Diabetes Acknowledgment

As I was preparing for my six-month follow-up appointment, I was as giddy as a schoolboy, knowing that I had exceeded the goals that my doctor had prescribed for me! After my evaluation, I was bursting with anticipation to hear the news that I had beaten my diabetic condition in just six months! But as the doctor started to explain, yes, my hard work was good, but he would not recommend ending the pills. Stopping the medication could be harmful to my overall health! So, I asked about his earlier statements about curing diabetes! This was the moment that this incurable sickness was a life sentence!

I continued to exercise and eat right, only to find out in future doctor visits that the pills were less and less effective in fighting my condition. Therefore, I was prescribed insulin injection therapy, morning shots, lunch shots, and night shots before bed. Through this method I quickly regained the weight that I had originally lost and gained much more than that. I was bloated, and so much of the weight was liquid weight as the years passed from age forty-five to fifty-five years old.

At the age of sixty, the veins in my legs became clogged, so I developed an ulcer on the bottom of my left foot. This incident was the first stage of failure of my left leg. I suffered six years of surgeries and skin grafts on my left foot and leg, including toe amputations, and finally the decision was to amputate the left leg below the knee!

Mentally, I was ready for the diseased portion of my body to be removed. A person must embrace adversity and move on from it! I reminisce about the journey from my first acknowledgment of having the dreaded "Sugar" and the cascading years of surgeries, trying to save a limb that was doomed to be replaced eventually. Yes, months and weeks would go by, and it seemed as if things were getting better, then I would wake up one day, and unexpectedly, I would realize that I was leaking fluids from a toe or there was another sore on top of the foot or bottom of the foot! Then another procedure to fix another problem, always thinking, when is this going to stop?

Religion

Growing up in the fifties and sixties, African Americans were emerging from years of abuse, depression, and violence, whether mental or physical. Families bonded under the spirit of a heavenly Father would lead us out of America's version of Egypt! The cry then and now is, "Lord, save us now or lift the veil that is covering our lives." Several gospel songs, like Singing the Blues Songs, were penned during these tumultuous times!

Examples:
"Lead Me, Guide Me, Oh Jehovah"
"God is Our Rock of Salvation"
"There Is a Storm Out in the Ocean"
"This Old Ship of Zion Shall Lead Me Home"
"The Battle Is Not Yours—It's the Lord's"

So, I had no choice but to trust in an invisible God and Jesus Christ. When times get tough in our home and family, work, or school life, prayer is the remedy! Somehow, the cosmic atmosphere would move on our behalf and things would be better, if not immediately, over time! It was always my belief that dreadful things and times do not work themselves out by themselves. You know a lot of people would say, "Son, just give your problems time, and they will work themselves out automatically." I doubted this philosophy very seriously! Our church, a Christian-based religion, always emphasized a greater and higher power than ourselves!

All throughout my life, I worked or served in the church, either as an usher, deacon, armor bearer, or volunteer on outreach committees, trying to share the power of God's grace! Therefore, when I was going through my trials and tribulations with my leg and foot, I strongly held to my religious teaching and beliefs to trust in the higher power of God.

Doctors, friends, and onlookers would privately or openly say, "Dwight is not going to make it!" I would say inside myself when I heard the whispers or rumors, "You do not know who is fighting for me! And yes, I will make it—and be better physically than before!"

This powerful force in the universe is called by many names spoken and unspoken: The Unmoved, the Mover, or Help in the Times of Trouble.

The question that rings through the annals of time was, "Is there anything that is too hard for our Holy God?"

If God could conquer the Egyptians, raise several people from the dead, including Jesus, and if He could cure the dreaded disease of leprosy, then surely, He can cure "the Sugar."

One analogy that I used throughout my recuperation was, "If you do the crime, then be prepared to do the time." And come out on the other end better for it. Experience is the master teacher.

I grew up in a traditional family with a two-parent household, four siblings, in Detroit, Michigan. In the 1960s no one in my immediate family group had "the Sugar." In 1990 my father was showing signs of diabetes, along with some memory loss. He had just retired after thirty-five-plus years of working at the General Motors factory in Detroit. My mother and father were both veteran auto factory workers. Mother retired 4–5 years after Dad retired, and Dad soon died of complications from diabetes, aka "the Sugar," whispered or spoken aloud. Dad was an avid league and semi-pro traveling bowler!

None of the four boys in our immediate family were ever labeled lazy people or "couch potatoes."

I assumed that the age of lazy young people arrived in the United States with the invention of PlayStation games and the ALL Everything INTERNET!

My post-secondary and college days after my college football-playing days and graduation, I started coaching at my alma mater, Knoxville College. I was popular among our alumni base during my playing days. The team won a couple of conference championships. I was one of the leaders on and off the field. I was part of the Student Government Association. On the field, I was a celebrated All-American football player and team captain.

I soon got engaged and married a young lady from the neighboring college in Knoxville, Tennessee; I was twenty-five years old. Then eventuality happened and we soon had two children, both boys. I was pleased. Then I had the opportunity to coach both my sons in three different sports from five years old: T-ball, football, and basketball. Also, teaching them to swim by the survival method. The Survival Method for swimming was to jump in—do your best, and please do not drown. If you keep your mouth shut, your chances of survival will be enhanced.

So as time went along and the years passed by, with one boy in middle school and one in high school, my days of coaching them were over! The schools had long-term coaches on staff who insisted that the boys did things their way only!

I joined a competitive traveling softball team, the Steeles Silver Bullets. As I rose to stardom at my position as a homerun hitter, I practiced for long hours on the art of hitting, I played for several different teams, played 2–3 nights a week in local leagues.

Yes, I was finally back in my comfort zone—performing at the highest level of sports/softball. My memory chords kicked back in, and my skills were only slightly diminished! After a few weeks of intense training, workouts, jogging, and batting practice, my engine was humming like a well-oiled machine!

My favorite tunes, played in my subconsciousness without thinking about them:

1) Queen: "We Are the Champions"
2) Bon Jovi: "Wanted Dead or Alive"
3) Bob Seger: "Turn the Page"
4) From the movie *Gladiator:* "Win the Crowd;" "I Will Show Them Something They Have Never Seen Before"

Are you not entertained?

Okay, yes, I acknowledged and accepted that I was a diabetic. I had "a Touch of the Sugar." For the next few years, I assumed that everything was okay. I was back on top athletically and well-respected in my beloved sport—softball. My family was doing well. Work was going extremely well. I was very satisfied with my church life and had lots of friends.

But, at times, I would notice memory loss, hesitation in

my speech, and stiffness in my legs. I was already diagnosed with neuropathy—the loss of feeling in my feet. That did not bother me at all. I was a door-to-door salesperson for a roofing company! But gradually, at sixty years old, fifteen years after first being diagnosed with "the Sugar," I was in and out of the foot doctor's office. I then found myself in and out of the hospital having several treatments—skin grafts for foot wounds that would not heal! Little snips of my toes were being cut to remove diseased portions little by little over the following 5–6 years. Near the end of this period, I did not have anything that resembled a foot! All I had was a stump! Yes, no toes, but I could still walk. I spent weeks, months at a time in the hospital for these procedures. I was determined to keep fighting against the "Sugar." This whole scenario took a great toll on my support team, especially my very supportive wife!

So finally, after four and a half futile years of trying to save my foot and lower left leg, I made the decision eagerly, with no apologies, to amputate the left leg below the knee. I was already prepared to lose it anyway, so the executioner came into the operating room with the chainsaw and did the dastardly deed! Amputation!

The war against "the Sugar" had taken a negative turn against me! "The Sugar" had won a long-fought battle. My body was relieved to call the retreat, and I threw up the proverbial white flag. My mind went back to my reading of the book *The Art of War*—sometimes opponents in a battle must lose or relent their position in order to regroup, reorganize, rethink their position!

Second Quarter

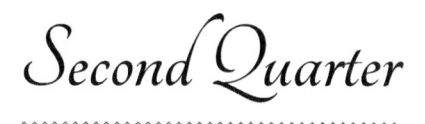

BISHOP KEVIN TREADWELL

SENIOR PASTOR

LEESBURG, VA

As the battle against the Sugar intensified, it was like a fast, high-scoring basketball or football game going into the second quarter.

The Power Of Consistent Prayer During Troubling Times

The scriptures tell us men should always pray and not faint (Luke 18:1). Prayer is very important for the Christian. Prayer is the power connection to God. The book of James, chapter 5:16b states, "The effectual fervent prayer of a righteous man availeth much." The believer should always pray, in the good times and during troubling times.

When we look at the Word of God and compare it to the times that we are currently living in, these could be troubling times. For example, there are diseases, pestilence, foodborne pathogens, wars, rumors of wars, earthquakes, hurricanes, and many people are being very deceitful.

Those who are in a right relationship with God can pray and expect results from God. There are many examples of Christians in troubling times who call upon the Lord in prayer and receive help from God. For instance, in 1 Samuel 7:8–10, when the children of Israel were fearful of the Philistines who were attacking them, the prophet Samuel prayed to God to help the children of Israel, and He interceded for them and defeated the Philistines.

The Bible is full of examples of the power of consistent prayer during troubling times. I have personally seen God answer my prayers many times when I was in a difficult situation. The scripture says in Psalm 46:1 that "God is our refuge and strength, a very present help in trouble."

The Bible holds the keys to the power of consistent prayer during troubling times. One key is found in the Gospel of John 15:7: "If ye abide in me, and my words abide in you, ye shall ask what ye will, and it shall be done unto you. That is the power of consistent prayer during troubling times."

BISHOP KEVIN L. TREADWELL
Leesburg, VA

The Verdict Was Cast

Man versus "the Sugar" and "the Sugar" won the battle.

The reality of being handicapped set in a few days after the amputation! I had to quickly come to terms with the fact that this was *permanent*. So, I lay in the hospital bed thinking positive as usual. How can this be a good thing? Several questions ran through my mind. Will I be in a wheelchair? Will I have to walk with a cane? Will I lose my other leg later on? Just think about the horror of being a double amputee! Gee Whiz!

I was lying there thinking of all my self-serving accomplishments. Now I will be relegated to back page news as a *has-been*—the once-popular high school legend and college football star. I could clearly see myself looking back at all of the home runs that I hit in the past!

The journey from stardom to amputee was a long, rocky, downward fall! Below are just a few of my tidbits of sports-related highlights:

1) High School All American
2) Three Sport Star in high school football, basketball, track

3) All-City Performer in basketball
4) All State Performer in football
5) College All-Conference Selection in football for three consecutive years
6) All-American in final senior season
7) Selected as a free agent with San Francisco (NFL)
8) And tryouts with the Dallas Cowboys and Atlanta Falcons
9) 5X All-American in softball during my career to this point

When you think about my vainness, playing sports was like a woman's hair in that a woman's hair is her glory—playing was my glory. Yes, losing my leg was the most devastating thing that ever happened to me—I would guess the same conclusion for a lot of people! In the midst of sulking in my new situation, I asked the doctor what was next. A little Greek podiatrist told me:

1) You can sit there and become a human vegetable with your wheelchair being your lifelong crutch.

2) You can determine your own future! You can get off your butt and endure the pain of walking again! DO IT NOW!

A Greek doctor, God bless his soul, told me I needed to get a rolled-up newspaper and beat my stump daily! I said what? Won't that hurt? Yes, it will, but you have to toughen up that remaining limb. So, I bought a newspaper or magazine and started the process of beating my stump daily!

I was referred to rehab therapy for 6–8 weeks. The therapist was amazed at how far along I was with movement, pain tolerance, and eagerness to improve and get out of rehab! I pressed my doctors to get me fitted for a prosthetic sooner than later!

After a long soul-searching inward reckoning, I vowed to continue to fight "the Sugar" with everything I've got!

After six months of rehabbing and learning how to manage life with a prosthetic leg, I began working out with light weights in a sitting position. I definitely did not have enough strength or dexterity to balance my body and lift weights!

In my youthful, joyous days, I was a workout phenom. I could bench press 450 pounds, leg press 1,000 pounds, do 100-pound standing hammer curls, and do regular curls at 150 pounds. Reverse curls, I could do pull downs with all the weight on the machine. So that very night, looking through tear-stained eyes from self-pity, my comeback plan was hatched and cemented. In my inner sanctum, I would survive and thrive through these devastating effects of "the Sugar," aka diabetes. I attended church in a wheelchair, but I gradually moved to using a walker to get around!

Then as I progressed through rehab therapy, I graduated to a walking cane! I never got used to moving around with traditional crutches! So, after several months of rehab, I was placed on a beginner's prosthetic. It was heavily padded and awkward, clumsy. I often was afraid of falling and breaking a hip or arm!

I felt helpless, like a newborn babe. I needed my wife's help with getting in and out of bed, getting into the bathroom, showering, cooking meals. It was extremely frustrating just to get in and out of our car, which luckily was an SUV.

Remember the old saying that you do not miss a body part until you do not have it? If you ever wondered what it would be like to be blind or paralyzed or how you could operate with one arm or one leg, one eye, or to be deaf. It is not fun! Re-learning how to do things is hard!

Why Is Forty-Five The Magic Age For Diabetes?

I was sailing along through life, being not overly concerned with others, avoiding strife and stress. I was being blessed and faithful in the eyes of our Lord and Savior, Jesus Christ! So, I was totally caught off guard when I started suffering the effects of "the Sugar." I often asked, "Lord, why me?" I am one of the good guys, so I thought! Then I took the self-pity veil off my eyes and remembered my religious teaching that trouble comes to the saved and unsaved. It is just a matter of how you react to trouble when it comes your way!

What Are The Early Symptoms Of Diabetes?

Acknowledged or ignored, below are some signs of being touched with "the Sugar." Being touched seems morbid, like being a person with leprosy in the Bible, which was incurable. That is why there is a lot of fear and trepidation when "the Sugar" comes knocking at your door!

Yes, a lot of us were hoping that "the Sugar" was just coming to visit for a few days, like a bad cold, hypertension, or dehydration. You know the prescription is usually light medication and several days of rest! Humorously, you know when "the Sugar" makes a house call, it is coming for more than just an overnight or weekend visit among family and friends! "The Sugar" has an agenda: its plan is for permanency at your house!

Okay, one of my signs of the dreaded Sugar was that I was urinating a lot more than normal. Secondly, as previously stated, I started losing weight, and I was not trying. Yes, I was running—more like light jogging—working out in the gym, swimming, and playing lots of softball. My energy level was dropping. I was getting fatigued quicker. I attributed this to summer heat and weight loss. No Big

Deal! So, I thought. But the symptoms doubled. Then tripled. In some instances, my vision got blurry. Then I got worried! I asked myself if my vision changes were an aging thing. I started cramping more in my legs. This was not normal since I was a thirty-plus-year athlete at forty-five!

Climbing Up The Rough Side Of The Mountain To Full Recovery

One of my favorite Bible verses is Philippians 3:13: "I do not count myself to have apprehended: But this one thing I do, forgetting those things which are behind and reaching forward to those things which lie ahead!" This verse addresses my situation very well to a T.

Let me explain. Diabetes did not happen to me by accident; I have a family bloodline that made me pre-diabetic, and I myself played a pivotal role in enhancing the effects of "the Sugar." I had an insatiable appetite for sweets. I could consume massive quantities of sweets.

Therefore, a couple of years ago, I began to see light at the end of the rehab tunnel. I would go out to the ballpark to practice hitting. I was like a stick man—standing straight up and down—not much of any flexibility. The pitcher would throw me a pitch; the best I could do was to hit it lightly or softly back towards him or over to the first base side of the infield.

As time went on, I began hitting softballs over the second baseman's head, realizing that I was an extremely powerful hitter in my pre-sugar issues days. Now I was just a shell of myself! The guys in the league that I played in were kind enough to let me play! I could not run, just walk fast! So, they agreed to let me hit and someone else would run from home plate for me!

At the level of mobility that I was at, I could only use my arms to swing the bat. I still did not have proper movement of power in my lower body and not full control of the prosthetic leg. I, therefore, planned for the next season. I would begin working my lower body in the health spa. Then I would go to the swimming pool three days a week! Just like a blinded Hercules, I felt my strength returning four years post-amputation! During my batting practice days, I started hitting balls again toward the left side of the field! I felt blessed just to be able to be sixty years old and play the game that I loved so much! The next season, I hit a home run or two in the first couple of league games. The other guys quickly said it was not fair for me to have a runner running for me, and all I had to do was hit!

So, we had some heated discussions! The result of the discussions was that I had to run for myself! But I stated that even though I could slowly run for myself, I am the same guy playing with prosthetic limbs. I soon became a show to younger "guys and girls" playing in the league! How can this sixty-something old man with one leg hit better than most of the players in the league! Someone called me an "enigma," meaning extra ordinary, puzzling, or amazing! Therefore, I count myself not lucky or to have apprehended. But by the grace of God, I was thriving from my past surgery, looking ahead to the future.

Lifelong Hospital Avoidance

There is a consensus that most men will avoid going to the hospital like it was the bubonic plague. Women, on the other hand, if they get a sneeze or a cough, they rush to see a doctor. So, the theory behind men avoiding doctors is that if you are not deathly sick, do not go. Therefore, once you go into the hospital, they start running a whole battery of tests. Men are afraid that if it seems like nothing is wrong with us, the doctor or hospital will find something wrong. We then heard all the rumors that once you go in the hospital for a simple knee operation, you may never come out again. These were the kind of tales that were told at all the barber shops throughout America. Everyone knows that barbers are experts at everything. Also, whatever is spoken in a barbershop or beauty shop is the "gospel truth," right? Some men still believe that the cow jumps over the moon every Halloween and that a 350-pound Santa Claus still comes down a narrow chimney with a bag full of gifts.

So as my experiences in the hospital and post-surgery issues continued to mount, I somehow picked up a blood infection, and I was prescribed antibiotics for six weeks. My first option was to stay in the hospital for six weeks while they administered the antibiotics via a PICC line. A PICC line is a peripherally inserted central catheter (PICC) line, which is a thin, flexible tube that is inserted into a vein in the upper arm and then advanced into the large central vein near the heart.

My second option was to go home and continue the treatment. I picked going home in a millisecond. I had already been in the hospital for two months. My thinking was, I just needed to get out of this place. I felt like the hospital was slowly sucking and draining the life out of me. Yes, in the back of my mind, I thought that the barbers at the corner barbershop were right. I might die in this place.

But my fears were laid to rest. The procedure of installing the PICC line was painless and I had to receive medication every day. At the same time, nightly, the nursing assistants showed my wife exactly how to administer the antibiotics. The key was cleanliness; yes, cleanliness was next to godliness. The blood infection happened at least twice over the six or seven years after the surgeries.

Work Environment—Work Ethic

I was always driven by the innate fear of failure. Let me say a few words about how "the Sugar" affected my work career as a fully commissioned sales manager.

I worked full time for the last eighteen years for my current employer. Sometimes I had to do door-to-door canvassing for potential roof replacement clients. With my intense work ethic firmly entrenched in my personality, I would work ten hours a day developing my craft at selling. I quickly became the annual sales leader at my company. I won several sales awards and bonuses! The game plan was easy! The harder you worked, the more you earned! This style of working suited me better than the typical 9–5 job!

Boy, did I like making money! A six-figure annual income allowed me and my family to live the American Dream on a moderate scale, of course! Then someone whispered, "Dwight has a 'touch of the Sugar.'" My wife and mother simultaneously screamed, "NO, NOT THE SUGAR."

I was accustomed to managing all my contracting deals with customers. Also, I enjoyed being on site when the jobs were being completed, and then the fun part—collecting the checks! As I stated previously, the first six months post "SUGAR" surgery, I was in a wheelchair and a walker! So, I could not drive, walk, climb stairs, etc.! I could still write contracts, but I needed someone to do the things that I used to do—satisfy customers.

The way it worked, I would pay referral fees to anyone that referred me to a friend, neighbor, co-worker, family member, mother, father, or ex-wife or ex-husband. It really did not matter to me! Even though I was in communication n via the telephone or the internet, bills still had to be paid. In the service industry, there is no real loyalty. If I could not satisfy the customer's immediate need right away, they would call someone else. I was not about to let that happen. No sir, not at my income level!

I had to pay most of my commissions to younger employees, just to make ends meet! Half the money was still better than no money! This was the main reason that I worked extra hard at getting on my feet as quickly as humanly possible!

As the weeks and months went by, I began to walk, although slowly, but I was back in the game! Doing my own contracting again, sitting in my truck overseeing roofing jobs and collecting checks! Yes, I did fall out of the #1 sales leader position for 2–3 years. But, like my sports involvement, my work career also began to "rise out of the ashes like a phoenix"

No, I am not the same hard-charging, ten-hour-a-day salesperson like I was in my "pre-sugar days." I learned, just like a lot of older professionals do when the world puts you out to pasture! The great Michael Jordan said he had to learn how to work smarter, not harder! Yes, I am truly on my way back in the "Game of Life."

How Can You Measure Pain?

Some measure pain on a sliding scale of intensity from 1 through 10, with 10 being the most intense.

Then the question is, how does one determine pain tolerance? Does everyone have the same level of pain tolerance? I can answer this question quite easily! *NO*. Most of my doctors, nurses, therapists, etc., stated that I had an extremely high tolerance for pain! Throughout the entire nine-year journey through the "SUGAR" operations cycle, I was noted as never flinching. Never complained openly about the pain, like most patients.

Let me tell you about the three worst ambulance rides.

Shortly after returning to work after an extensive stay at the hospital and weeks of rehabbing from one of my toe removal procedures, I was back driving my company truck. On my way from one sales appointment to another, I found myself sitting and waiting for what seemed to be like an hour in school zone traffic. Waiting in the truck with the gear set in park, the school crossing guard suddenly allowed the oncoming traffic to move. My truck was eight to ten vehicles back from the crossing guard area.

Suddenly, out of nowhere, a car came right at me! Missing the other nine cars, it hit me almost head-on! The impact flipped my truck over, and I landed upside down in it! Yes, the other vehicle hit me on the driver's side, and luckily, I was wearing my seat belt. I had to reason with the situation; I was upside down in my seat belt and the truck was running, so I first rolled my window down and released my seat belt. Then I turned the truck off and crawled out of the window. The driver's side door was crushed shut, but thank God, the electric window still worked—yes, thankfully the engine was still running while I lay there upside down. I heard my inner self saying, "Oh, God! Oh, God! Help me get out of this truck before it explodes or catches fire!"

I got out and found my work chair on a small two-lane road. I walked or hobbled over to pick it up. There I sat in my work chair at an accident scene next to my upside-down truck. The sheriff arrived and was amazed at how calm I was after being in a rollover accident while in the parked position. The officer called my job, and a co-worker attempted to reach my wife for me, thinking of a hysterical, loving wife. My belongings and phone were scattered on the road and inside the vehicle. A kind gentleman came over to check on me, and I asked to use his phone to call my wife. She told me she was running errands, saw the strange number, and returned the call; it was me.

When Rhonda arrived on the scene, I was still sitting in the chair next to the upside-down truck. The ambulance had just arrived, and the first responders were checking me for injuries. The only obvious injury was my newly amputated toes. I told them I was fine. They asked me to stand up, and I was whisked away to the local trauma emergency room. Let me make this clear: riding in an ambulance is a very, very painful ride. When I arrived at the emergency room, I was hurting worse than being in a head-on collision!

My second ride occurred while I was at the hospital on another occasion—the amputation of my big toe and another five-week stint in rehab. I would have to take an ambulance ride from the hospital to the rehab center, which was right around the corner. Trust me, these rides were brutal. I almost said, "Lord, I would have been better off walking!" But of course, I could not because I had had major surgery and had only a foot with no toes.

The last ambulance ride of my ongoing saga! As I stated in earlier chapters, everything would be going along like peaches and cream, then I would wake up from a good sleep and there would be blood everywhere around the remaining portion of the foot. Yes, it was just a stump without toes. My wife received a call from our daughter, who is an LPN. She shared what was happening and told my wife to call an ambulance immediately. I was rushed to the first hospital emergency room of my choice, only to be told I needed to go to another hospital. After getting bounced around on this final ambulance ride, the doctor and I agreed that if the foot or leg did not kill me, the ambulance ride would! Each time I would endure these painful ambulance rides or excursions, I would ask the question, "Lord, how long will this trouble go on?" The answer would always be the same… "My Grace is Sufficient."

Hospital Vampires

There were several occasions when I went to follow-up medical check-up appointments. I was pre-surgery scared of needles being injected into my veins; currently, I must admit, after literally hundreds of injections by nursing assistants and pre-surgery anesthesiologists sticking me, I am not as scared or fidgety. Finding my veins became more and more mysterious or elusive as my diabetes intensified.

Most people do not understand the difference between drawing blood samples and setting up an intravenous line. As young athletes, we were encouraged to donate blood to the Red Cross and other life-saving agencies. Some friends would sell their plasma for about fifty dollars at the local blood bank. Fifty dollars for a struggling college student was good money to sustain you until your care box from home arrived at the dorm. I was not a fan of the process of selling my blood or plasma. Yet, I would do my civic duty to help others.

Back to my fear or avoidance of needles of any kind on different occasions. Newer nursing or surgery assistants seemed like they were in stick-a-vein training. It would take them several attempts to find a vein to draw blood from or set up an IV line. I eventually identified the nurses as vampires. These attempts were extremely painful. The nurse would have to beat or thump my arm so that the vein would pop up or show itself to the so-called vampire; the nurse would go from arm to arm in search of a vein.

Then, setting up an IV line that would stay in the arm for days or weeks at a time was another issue. This line would be placed on the back of my hand, a highly sensitive area, as a portal to provide needed IV fluids and medications. The back of the hand is mainly constructed of bones and veins, whereas when drawing blood, the inner middle part of the arm is constructed of lots of meaty flesh and muscle and then veins. So, if there is an injection miss, it hurts but not as much. With the injection portal on the back of the hand, it was taped down to my skin so that it would not come out during the night when I was asleep and while tossing and turning through the night.

Please, do not let anyone tell you that hospital beds are comfortable because they are not. Also, do not let them tell you that being in the hospital is like going on vacation for two weeks or two months at a time. Yes, during my hospital stay, I once told the attending nurse or charge nurse to just take a sharp knife and cut my veins at the wrist and collect my blood that way—it is a lot easier than this trial-and-error method that is being applied to my veins. But they do their best and are only human too.

Common Cliques

Where your heart is, is where your fears and energy will be.

Life has its ebbs and flows.

I cannot just fish from the sheltered shore. I must go out into the deep sea where the big fish are.

Even though all death is certain! You control most of your own destiny.

The pain relief of choice is morphine. Morphine: The Happy Drug.

Leg and foot pain is extremely painful. The human body has located all of, or most of, the nerve endings down through the legs to the foot.

Some studies show that a lot of leg amputee patients never get out of the wheelchair after surgeries! Whether it is a single or double amputation, there is no true rhyme or reason. It could be because of extremely low pain tolerance, mental or physical reasons, or they just simply gave up on being seen as a whole person again, so why bother? It seems easier for someone else to worry about you and tend to all your needs, like driving, washing, clothing you or bathing you, and cooking for you, than trying to do it yourself!

I personally know of individuals who could not even bear to be touched. They could not withstand the wind blowing too hard. So, this is one of the reasons that I was labeled "an enigma" for having an extremely high pain tolerance. But as a reminder, my pain relief drug of choice was morphine! I called it the Happy Drug.

With this drug, I would have it injected, and within a few seconds I would be off into never-never land! I would wake up five or six hours later and eat lunch or dinner! The attending nurses would say, "Do you want to watch TV or get another dose of morphine?" You can already guess what my answer was!

Yet, once I would leave the hospital after certain procedures, I would only take Tylenol and endure minor levels of pain!

So, I was determined to get out of the wheelchair and walkers, and eventually walked with the assistance of a cane! Lots of people told me that I was working too fast, moving forward too quickly. My answer was, "I cannot fish at the sheltered shore! I must go out into the deep sea to catch the Big Fishes in Life."

This quote was something I enjoyed! Requoting it became one of my favorites.

Throughout my life and even now, I vowed to never become a legendary "couch potato!" The Bible talks about two lepers hiding out in the mountains observing a great battle forming down below! They said to themselves, "We can sit here and starve to death, or we can get up and go down to the valley where there is food and live!"

Fellow Amputees—I encourage you, if at all possible, to endure the pain or whatever obstacle that might be holding you back from getting out of that wheelchair crutch and living your best life! Yes, of course, different pain relief prescriptions are better for your pain than mine! Your doctor is the best source for pain management. I am not advocating that you do what I did. But maybe realize when you start that your body will fight you to stay sedated, lethargic, and comfortable. Yes, changes in daily rituals and habits are not comfortable! Progress and growth are definitely not comfortable or easy.

Halftime

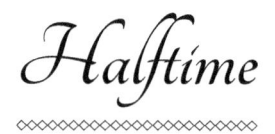

PASTOR ALBERT BRY, JR.
SENIOR PASTOR
SECOND AVENUE BAPTIST CHURCH
BIRMINGHAM, AL
Defensive Coordinator

Well, this is like a team that was favored to win by two touchdowns and found themselves down forty to zero. In the locker room, much soul-searching is done about what has gone wrong and what corrective actions need to be taken.

Spiritual Preparation For What's Yet To Come

When I was a student at Briarwood Theological Seminary, Dr. Thad James, professor of Biblical Interpretation, had a daily mantra that was repeated at the beginning of every class that went like this: "proper preparation prevents poor performance." There was another "p" that came before poor, but I will leave that to your imagination. The emphasis was on being prepared for class as well as the various assignments that came along with the course.

Such is the case with life in general, but more importantly, spiritually. From a general perspective, most of us have thought about how to prepare for storms. Perhaps we've seen and or felt the suffering of women, men, and children, young or aged, weak or strong, caught in the throes of tornados, hurricanes, tsunamis, wars, and droughts. The fact of the matter is that not all storms are alike. Not all storms are created equal. Storms vary in form and in severity.

The question then becomes, "How can I be prepared?" Do I go out in a rush to purchase and stockpile whatever it is that I think I might need for the day when I may face such tragedies? That is the general perspective.

There is another even more important preparation we must make for tests that are certain to come to each of us, for Jesus forewarns us in John 16:33 (TLB), "Here on earth you will have many trials and sorrows." What we will need on our day of testing is the most important preparation: spiritual preparation.

Blackaby states, "There is no substitute for spiritual preparation. Spiritual preparation equips you for unforeseen crises or opportunities. However, if you are unprepared, you will be vulnerable in life's unexpected events."[1]

Spiritual preparation must be started far in advance because it takes time. It takes time to spend time alone with God. It takes time to pray, meditate, and study the Word, Works, and Wonders of God. It is within the discipline of spiritual preparation that you developed a faith in Jesus Christ, a faith that can't be bought or borrowed; however, it does store well and must be used frequently and daily, a faith in Jesus Christ so powerful that you can stand as well as pass the tests of life, which are certain to come. It is in spiritual preparation that you acquire what you need in order to survive the trials, sorrows, and storms of life.

To spiritually prepare is to practice spiritual discipline.

Preparation and discipline are a perfect pair of virtues for the child of God, who seeks to be victorious over the adversities of life.

As a former athlete, I am very familiar with the process of preparation and discipline. Both of those practices in the sports arena have also aided me in the spiritual arena of life. Besides the commonality of the two, I would argue that preparation and discipline are most valuable in the offseason.

In the sports arena, the offseason is defined as a time of year when a particular sport is not engaged. It is during the offseason that preparation and discipline have their greatest value.

It is in the offseason that an athlete must be disciplined enough to prepare on his or her own. Disciplined enough to eat right on their own. Disciplined enough to work out on their own. Disciplined enough to get the proper rest on their own. All of these things take place during the season, but the difference is that you have a dietician making sure you eat right. You have a trainer making sure you train right. You have a coach that enforces curfews to make sure you rest right. Again, I argue that it is in the offseason that you prepare and discipline yourself for both adversity and victory.

Likewise, the offseason in the spiritual life is one of the most valuable times for the child of God. The offseason in the spiritual arena is that time of praying without being made to but because you love to. The offseason in the spiritual arena is that time of fasting, not because of some dilemma, but because I am disciplined enough to live a disciple's life. The offseason in the spiritual arena is that time of feasting and meditating upon the Word of God before the season of failing health, relationships, finances, and so many other circumstances and situations that leave us with no other alternative but to call on the name of the LORD.

It is when we're disciplined and prepared in the offseason that we will be able to handle both the adversity as well as the victory that seasons of life bring.

Practical Application of Spiritual Preparation, and Thus, Spiritual Discipline

Spend time alone with God by way of:

1. Prayer—develop a consistent prayer life.

2. Meditation—saturate your mind and heart with the Word of God.

3. Praise—cultivate an attitude that will bless the LORD at all times, in the offseason as well as during the various seasons of life.

Those are just a few to help you spiritually prepare for what is yet to come.

Pastor A.W. Bry Jr.
Victory Missionary Baptist Church
706 SECOND Avenue North Birmingham, Alabama 35203

You Do Not Need Medical Training To Be An At Home Caregiver

A lot of spouses and partners have this heavy burden of making a mistake that will cause harm to the patients. Through our in-home experiences, my caregiver, Rhonda, had to change wound bandages and administer intravenous (IV) antibiotic drugs through my arm on two separate occasions after leaving the hospital!

We were given sanitary practices instructions that were easy to follow, like washing hands, wearing gloves, wearing a mask, closing one valve to add new medicines, re-opening valves to allow drug flow, and proper disposal.

My Caregiver's Point Of View

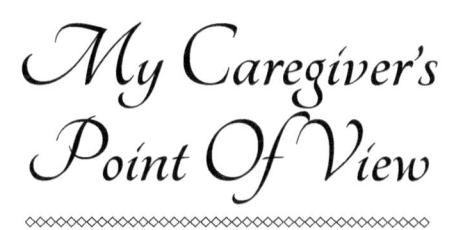

June 22, 2014, is a day I will never forget. It began a ten-year journey I will never regret.

My husband, Dwight "Tread" Treadwell, was complaining about his left foot a few days earlier. I, of course, suggested he see a doctor and reached out to my brother-in-law, who suggested he come in and see him. Well, you have to understand my husband. He is always "busy" and did not make that appointment. On that fateful Saturday morning, the foot was swollen, and he said, "Let us go to Campbell Clinic." I had been there several times due to arthritis in my knee, and we assumed it was a bone that had been injured. Boy, were we wrong! Once we checked in, and while waiting to be called back to see a doctor, the swollen foot popped and the smell was, let me say, extremely unpleasant, and I immediately said to myself, "We are in the wrong place."

Once the doctor saw us, he immediately stated that we needed to go directly to the hospital, and the closest one was Methodist Germantown. We entered the emergency room, and with the call from the doctor at the clinic, we were placed in an observation room. This doctor examined him and asked the nurse to prep him for emergency surgery. The interesting thing about this particular day was that he was the only patient there. The anesthesiologist was available, as well as the surgeon, and they took him in immediately.

After an hour of surgery, the doctor came to me, and I already knew what he was about to tell me. I asked, "So what is going on?" And he said my husband was going to lose his foot and leg. I, in turn, said, "It is deadly?" And he said, "Yes." I told him to go ahead and do what was necessary to save his life. His response was, "No, we need to evaluate the actual cause of the issue," and he explained it is like peeling an onion—we must remove each layer to get to the cause.

Tread was admitted within two hours and for the next four weeks I watched his foot die.

I first called both our pastors, who came and prayed with us and for us. I notified his mother and siblings; my immediate family was already aware. I requested no visitors because I could not answer any questions, and the foot was exposed and open. It was safer to not have any visitors due to the nature of his open wound to cut down on infection. The doctor later told me that I had made the best decision.

The first week was like we were in a luxury hotel, with excellent service and attention from the doctors, nurses, hospital techs, etc. The attending surgeon said he needed to inject dye into the leg to determine the circulation issues—the foot was not getting blood. Without blood flow, the foot was slowly dying. There were concerns about injecting the dye and the effect it would have on his kidneys, but after two weeks, the procedure was done. We were referred to an interventional radiologist who roto-rootered the veins and arteries in the leg. It was determined that veins needed to be taken from the right leg to restore blood flow in the left leg. This procedure included skin grafts and overall, it was successful.

Once the first surgery was complete, I was never so happy in my life to see the dying foot actually bleeding. It was later determined that another surgery was necessary to determine what level of loss would be of his foot. There was no guarantee that the foot could or would be saved. This was the fourth visit to the operating room, and I was anxious, truly uncertain as to whether or not the foot was to be completely removed or not. I got the call from the recovery room that he was out of surgery and would be returning to the room in an hour or so. He was taken back to the room and was semi-awake and completely covered from head to toe. After the attendant left, I pulled back the covers and found that he still had his foot!

Now, during these weeks, I was working full time as an operations manager of a new telephone call center. I was responsible for fifteen A-type millennial supervisors, all under the age of twenty-four, and 350 call center workers on a 12 a.m.–11 p.m. shift. This required I go to the hospital by 7 a.m. each morning and report to work no later than 9 a.m. Leave on my lunch break to check in with Tread at the hospital and return to work until 11:30 p.m.

Now my husband was a perfect patient. Throughout the entire time in the hospital, not one time did he complain, whimper, or express any discomfort. Each day we prayed and thanked God for that day, the doctors, nurses, and anyone who came in contact with him during the day. His mother came to visit and spent twenty-one days with us while he was in the hospital, and she became his personal physical therapist.

Because Mother was there, I could not stay in the hospital with him; therefore, each evening we would get dinner, go home, sleep, and get back up and return to the hospital. I bathed him daily and made sure the room was clean and comfortable. I have a low threshold for waiting on others to address my loved ones' personal needs when I could do it myself. After twenty-one days, Mom had to return home. Her stay was a true blessing to both of us, and to be honest, Tread and his mother have a special bond through their faith in God and belief in attending church.

To say I was an emotional wreck is an understatement, but never did I ever share my tears or heavy heart with Tread or in his presence. I held my emotions until I got home alone and prayed and cried myself to sleep. I had to show strength and confidence and have a level head to communicate with the medical staff. Mind you, I also addressed all the needed functions at home—paying the bills, watering the flowers. Tread loves to see things grow and had planted flowers and fruit trees. Now we were in the dead of July, the hottest part of the summer, and I could not just leave his work undone.

God is ever so amazing because throughout this entire time, I wanted for nothing nor needed anything, and that which I did need was provided. Faith, hope, and, more importantly, gratitude were my stronghold. I thank God for everything—good, bad, and indifferent. By the end of our stay at the hospital, it seemed as though we were downgraded as far as luxury was concerned. The actual surgeon who had done the surgery was on vacation when it was time for us to leave.

The attending doctor stated, "Oh, I remember you. I advised the surgeon not to save your foot." The attending nurse said, "You must be coming from the Med, which is the only time I have seen a procedure like this."

I was completely insulted by both of them, but the positive aspect was that we were being released to the rehabilitation facility just around the corner.

Tread was released from the rehabilitation hospital on August 2. We planned for a Sunday school member to sit with him while I was at work; there were physical therapy home visits, IV antibiotics, scheduled doctors' appointments, and more. But on August 5, I was called into the new operations manager's office and was told my services were no longer needed. I smiled and said, "Thank you!" They looked at me strangely! I had to collect some of my personal items and leave the premises. This was a blessing for sure because I needed to be at home with Tread. Losing my job was just what we both needed. So, the real joke was on them.

After a month or so, Tread and I were in a well-oiled routine, and although we were not strained financially, it was unfair that I was not getting unemployment benefits. So, one day I went online and attempted to report my claim; I did this three times, and each time the computer screen went blank. Later that week, I received a call from the State inquiring about my firing.

Well, by this time, there was not much to say or tell them. Four days later, I received a text message from the HR director informing me that my benefits would not be denied. He explained that my work and my presence were of value. The company had determined this new guy would be hired, and I kept things up and running until he was able to relocate to Memphis.

Tread went on his first doctor's visit. By this time, we had the wheelchair, the shower had been converted so that it was more handicap accessible, and we had a wound vac. Crutches were highly uncomfortable for him, so we got a walker.

We had not been to church in over eight weeks, and we were armor bearers. We sat on the front row at the church. A church member came by to visit, and we asked if anybody was holding that station or sitting in those seats while we were out, and her response was, "No, no one is or has occupied those seats." Instead, everyone was just waiting for us to return.

Following the doctor's visit and once we got home, Tread said to me, "If I can go to a doctor's appointment, I can go to church. Hey, take me to the barbershop so I can get a haircut. I want to go to church on Sunday."

Our return to church on that Sunday was, well, words cannot describe. We had both lost weight and were just so happy to be back in corporate worship. You see, I never missed a week of paying our tithes. We continued to respond to family and friends to just pray with us and for us. Tread got his strength and confidence back.

The next phase was to have another visit with the interventional radiologist, who made sure the blood in the left leg was flowing properly to his foot. By this time, I was concerned about the right leg, but the doctors were more focused on the left leg for now.

I became his feet and legs. Funny thing, Tread never stopped actually working. You see, my husband is in sales, and each week when he was in the hospital, he was getting a paycheck. We are now a true sales team. My husband was in the minority yet was continually the highest grossing in sales.

What Happens When Your Caregiver Gets Sick?

Caregiving support is in itself not an easy job! It's vitally important that the caregiver takes the same number of precautions and care of themselves because they are the lifeline to the patient!

Like the marriage slogan: Happy Wife—Happy Life.

Caregiver Slogan: Happy Caregiver—Healthy Patient, and both survive the temporary setback!

The Caregiver, Historical Account Of "The Sugar" Making A House Call

On June 22, 2014, I rushed my husband to Germantown Methodist Hospital. He immediately went into surgery. Following the surgery, the doctor shared with me that he would lose his foot and leg. I asked if this would kill him, and the doctor said yes. But he shared that more investigation needed to be done. He used the example of peeling an onion, removing the layers to get to the cause of the issue. This was the beginning of our seven-week journey of hospital stay that included good and bad doctors, nurses, CNAs, janitors, staff, tech, etc.

My personal and emotional state was like this; here is the backstory:

April 2014—I accepted a new position.

June 2014—Dwight was into emergency surgery and was admitted into the hospital.

August 2, 2014—Dwight was released from the rehabilitation hospital. Note: the foot and left leg were saved.

August 5, 2014—I was fired from the new job/became

stay-at-home, full-time caregiver.

June 2019—After four and a half years, the final surgery was set; we were to have plastic surgery on the foot, and it would be supported in his shoe with an insert. Unfortunately, he contracted an infection, and instead of plastic surgery, we had a below-the-knee amputation.

Wow, it has been ten years! Who would have thunk it?

There are clearly several pain relief products on the market. As stated earlier, I was fearful of the strong pain relievers, like morphine, hydrocodeine, and others. A friend of my caregiver wife, Warren Chambers, called and said he had been working in the pain relief products industry! I said yes, that I would like to try some rather than keep using the "highly addictive" strong painkillers! He shipped me a box of five different creams, ointments, bath soaks, and sprays. I liked them all, but especially the magnesium-based pain relief rub-on cream.

Warren and I, over the years, developed a bond. He was looking for a distributor in Memphis, Tennessee. I am located in Memphis, so my wife, Rhonda, agreed to represent his products. Now we are owners of our distributorship called Nature's Best arthritis and muscle pain relief products.

After my surgery, I have arthritis flare-ups in my

hands. So, I used the massage cream extensively! A lot of post-surgery patients also noticed that they also have arthritis in various parts of their bodies. Just another example of "thriving" after suffering from "THE SUGAR."

Traveling Around The U.s.

At the age of twenty-nine, I was selected to play on a highly skilled softball team called the Steele's Silver Bullets, also known as "The Men of Steele." We traversed the continental USA by bus or van, traveling from state to state, playing local all-stars every night, two or three weeks at a time. This lasted about two years or so.

In my business career, I was a consultant to the Department of Energy out of Oak Ridge, Tennessee. Our group traveled to every Department of Energy site, talking and organizing public meetings. This travel was by plane, along with rental cars and weeklong hotel stays. I traveled over a million miles during this ten-year period. During these plane rides, on commercial planes like Delta, Northwest, and United American, the only adverse symptoms I noticed was my feet would swell up! I attributed it to the pressure from being 35,000 feet up in the air and the pressured cabins. Also, my eyes would pop because of the pressure of the cabin. Then after landing, the feet swelling reverted back to normal and the stuffy ears would clear up!

How Important Is The Support Of Your Spouse/The Caregiver

When the husband or the wife suffers a catastrophic injury, surgery, or malady, like a stroke or heart attack, it really does not matter if the situation was preplanned or accidental. Adversity, bad luck, bad timing—even death—is never ever convenient to the family structure. In most cases, the entire recovery of the patient is not convenient! The spouse or partner, in most cases, has a little more stress placed upon them than the actual injured partner. The spouse/caregiver does more direct lifting, dressing, washing, tucking, sleeping, wiping up, and cleaning private parts, and must also have an open ear for griping! Honey, can you do this or that for me!

The Spouse-Partner Caregiver

The non-injured caregiver has to be even-tempered. He or she cannot lose their temper if they get upset and mad at the injured. This attitude could send the injured one's recovery in a downward tailspin. The injured in 75 percent of households are still in a state of denial. Questioning, "Why did this happen to me? You have always caused me bad luck! Nothing good ever happens to me." The spouse/partner/caregiver in many cases is still working full or part time. And having to deal with all the challenges they face at work! Then come home and deal with a helpless, injured lifetime spouse! Immediately start dinner and put a load of clothes in the washer.

The caregiver has the entire weight of the household on his or her shoulders. The caregiver may even feel like they need counseling, just a break! It does not in most cases seem like progress, like the process is not moving fast enough!

Prayer and being able to talk with someone on the outside can be good for the soul! Even while they are giving constant encouragement to the injured, the caregiver may need encouragement themselves! Then late at night, when the house is quiet, everyone is fed, all the homework problems are solved, the caregiver can steal away to their special place, relax, and take a long sigh of relief.

At these special times they can hear their pastor say, "Do you take this person for better or for worse, in sickness and in health, for richer or poorer till death do you part?" These words somehow ring true in their subconscious! They will wind up jumping at every bump, cough, toe tap, slight sleepiness, elevated temperature, or slightly elevated blood pressure. They rush to the doctor's office or emergency room only to hear, "It's okay." The body is recalibrating itself.

Cliques

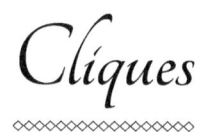

"America is a vast ocean of opportunities." —Dr. Martin L. King

What lies ahead for sufferers of "the Sugar?" What are my options for healthy living? Is it avoidance therapy, where you avoid sugar products, alcohol, starch, high-glucose substitutes, and milk by-products?

Can the normal person survive by only consuming natural products, unpasteurized, with no preservatives, no chemically enhanced fruits, vegetables, and meats, fowl, or fish? No, our bodies were created and designed to deal with and process all of the above! The problem sometimes is overindulgence or consuming too much of the wrong thing. But America's call to fame is a contributing factor to some of our health problems.

"America, land of the free, home of the brave." Does this statement or mantra mean to do what you want to do—consume as much as you can? In the old days, people were hunter-gatherers or farmers!

Now machines do a lot of labor-intensive duties, thanks to the onslaught or creation of automation and cybernation! This change in American evolution decreased our opportunities for exercise, either from working or recreation, and our immune systems have become compromised!

The body, once again, was created for motion. It has its own chemical warfare against what one ingests, consumes, or eats in an abundance of norms! But the defense is only activated when the body is in motion! Therefore, consume moderately in our vices, walk, run, skip, hop, dance, jump, swim, climb, ski, hike, join a team, start a league—something that fits your lifestyle or body type.

For older citizens who retire, studies conclude that the change in an active daily routine is a shock to the body's chemical warfare and leads to stagnation. Also, being solitary, stationary, relaxed, non-active, or having new routines confuses the internal systems. It is similar to adding too much pressure to a pipe that is clogged. The pipe is going to burst, slowly leaking bacteria and other internal stabilizers, which are then sent into the wrong areas of your body. And the next thing we know, "THE SUGAR," or cancer, stroke, heart attacks, lupus, vein blockages, etc., etc.

Therefore, my conclusion is to eliminate or decrease sugar. Limit overindulgence and a sedentary, lethargic lifestyle—stay active! This is only my opinion, fellow amputees. There is a place for us in this new age. There is always a need for volunteerism at schools, church, with veterans, work from home companies—our minds are still able to offer valuable services or resources to our society!

Release the demons and doldrums that feed negative, depressed self-worth!

The Second Half

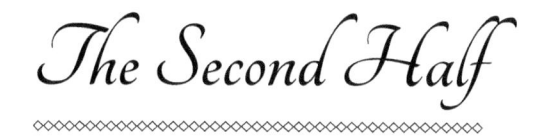

Elder Martin T. Treadwell Sr.

Former Pastor of Every Word Church

Detroit, Michigan, USA

Well, after a great halftime or intermission speech, action is required immediately, as it was in ancient times and as it is in modern times. Also, miracles in sports still occur, and miracles in sickness, disability, and all kinds of maladies still occur.

As believers, we are an incredibly blessed people. Why? I am glad you asked. Because God has promised in His Word: "For he hath said, I will never leave thee, nor forsake thee" (Hebrews 13:5). Therefore, a believer is endowed with the knowledge and privilege of knowing that God Almighty is ready and able to intervene in their lives at any time. Now, that is what I call a miracle.

A miracle is the manifestation of the power and presence of God doing what no other power can do. He does it instantly and openly, showing Himself in miracles whenever we are faced with or threatened with sickness, disease, unbelief, fear, or any curse or attack of the enemy, including the wiles of the devil. We know a miracle can show up at any time, whenever and wherever God pleases. In the book of Psalms it is recorded, "God is our refuge and strength, a very present help in trouble" (Psalm 46:1). "So that we may boldly say, the Lord is my helper, and I will not fear what man shall do unto me." (Hebrews 13:6). Therefore, believers qualify as candidates for miracles at any time.

Our God is faithful. He is the one true and living God; hence, He is fully committed to keeping His Word, and thus He watches over His Word to perform it. The Lord keeps His promises every day and graciously intervenes in the lives of His people to perform miraculous, marvelous miracles. The Lord works so seamlessly on our behalf, performing miracles that we can easily take for granted, though there are innumerable things that He does. God's Amazing Grace, His miracles, happen right at the appointed time, in time, and always on time.

We believers are the recipients of countless numbers of miracles seen and unseen. However, I have personally experienced the extraordinary power of God in my life in events too wonderful to completely explain. Events that have surpassed human understanding and explanation that can only be described as acts of divine intervention or the manifestation of God's power acting on my behalf, a miracle.

In conclusion, I am a walking, talking miracle of God. The Lord's miracles have stepped into my life on the job as a Detroit police officer for more than twenty-six years; God has kept me. As a husband and father, God has kept me. As a fisherman wading in the water, God has kept me. As a preacher of the gospel in God's pulpit, God has kept me. As a motorcyclist riding my motorcycle in traffic and getting hit by a car and lived, God has kept me.

I am a living testimony of the miracles that happen to regular people every day. For I am a recipient of God's miracles, His daily activity taking place every day, in all places, in people's lives everywhere. Glory of God. Amen.

Looking Forward To Your Future

Will your family remember you as the one who had the "TOUCH OF THE SUGAR" and gave up? Did you say in your time of weakness, "I will wait for a more opportune time. I need more information before I move. This thing could set me back too far. It will work itself out by itself, 'praying and fasting.'" Only time will be the great equalizer. But time is neutral. It can work for you or against you. Lastly, you might say my therapist is moving me too fast!

I say that if you are brave enough to start, you will not be remembered by these words: would of, could of, should of, loosely translated as "woulda, coulda, shoulda."

Yes, there are countless stories of individuals who overcame horrible accidents, devastating injuries, life-threatening sudden illnesses. This book serves only as encouragement for overcoming and thriving post-surgery. It details how active I was at work, in sports, at church, and with family!

Like a river, I had my high tides and low tides. But I did not lie on the sandy beach forever. I decided it was time to build my own boat and ride the "Tides of Thriving" post-surgery.

I give all thanks and gratitude to my God, caregiver, family, friends, co-workers—everyone who supported me through devastation to thriving. I did it—you can do it!

Verification Of Information

In the beginning of the book and inside the front cover, I stated that the information presented about surviving and thriving is absolutely a true story. It is my story. I am not some ghostwriter in a faraway ivory tower, thousands of miles away, or a starving artist/writer working out of his mother's basement suite. Included in this book are actual pictures of the story about the devastating effect of "THE SUGAR" on my lower left leg and foot! Yes, Sugar/Sweet Sugar!!

Sorry if the photos are a little too gory for your taste in paperback form. I will also attach several photos in an electronic file for you to look at your own discretion! There will be a link to the eight-year, hard-fought war against "THE SUGAR," whether whispered or said aloud.

Post-Surgery Anecdotal Memories

1. Mother and Her Jewelry
2. Robot Leg
3. Image of Leg Growing Back
4. The Leg Lamp
5. Ghost Pains
6. In-Home Adjustment: Baby VS Adult

My mother came to help my wife, Rhonda, with my personal health care for twenty-one days. This visit was right after my first amputation of three toes on my left foot. The human body responds immediately when pain is inflicted on any part of the system. Therefore, amputation is immediately quantified as an extreme attack on the human body's responses when pain is inflicted on a part of this system. Therefore, amputation is qualified as an extreme attack on the human skeletal system. Pain sensors function as first responders to that site. Even though the actual incident site was the foot, the whole body was alerted by the sensors that pain was present or imminent. With the amputation, I was hurting all over my entire body!

Realizing that this was my first time in a hospital for a unique kind of surgery, I was afraid to move from one position to the next because of the pain. I needed help to wash and go to the bathroom. My wife and mother had to give me a bath in the bed. Rhonda and my mother both wore lots of jewelry, i.e., ring bracelets. They both came from extensive cleaning backgrounds, meaning they would clean everything! They would clean hard and long. Remember my pain; tolerance sensors were on high alert. When you mix in the hard, long cleaning up my body along with the jewelry on their hands and wrists, I felt like I was in a meat grinder; I had to call a "Come to Jesus" meeting of the minds with my two most loving and trusted health care providers, Mom and Rhonda, begging them to lighten up the pressure on the cleaning. I told them, "Hey, I am not running or working out every day; thus, I am not that dirty. Secondly, please take off the jewelry, guys. I am fragile." Conclusion—this was painfully funny!

The days just before the executioner was scheduled to commune with a chainsaw and remove my lowly below-the-knee, I was dreaming about my favorite holiday movie, *The Christmas Story*. The main character was named Richie, and of course, it was only a movie, but the funniest part was when Richie's father ordered a leg lamp from an anonymous catalog. When it arrived at the house, he rearranged all the furniture in the living room so that he could put this prized possession front and center so the entire neighborhood could see it from his front living room window during the Christmas holidays.

The wife and kids hated that awful lamp, but the husband would not relent or be dissuaded from adoring the leg lamp. Then, one day, the family DOG got caught up in the wires to the leg lamp, and it broke. The husband was sorely disappointed as his holiday was suddenly ruined, yet he valiantly tried to glue and tape it back together but to no avail. The wife, Richie, and a little brother secretly laughed at the fact that the hideous leg lamp was broken. So, I was dreaming when they cut off my lower left leg that I could save it and make it into a leg lamp for the holidays! Just a humorous thought.

A year or so after the amputation, I would joke with my grandsons, who live in Nashville, Tennessee, that if I watered my remaining stump every day, it would grow. They would often ask if the leg had grown back, and I would say it is getting green.

A couple of years ago, Rhonda and I met our sons and grandson in Myrtle Beach, South Carolina. Our grandson is named after his father, William Carter Treadwell, Jr. He was five years old at the time of this visit and, to our knowledge, had never seen a prosthetic leg before. One morning, while at the pool, I took off my pants to change into my swimming shoes. William looked in amazement, his eyes bulging out of his head, with his mouth wide open, he shouted, "Paw Paw has a robot leg like on TV!" After calming down, he asked, "Can I touch it?" So, yes, some people will be shocked or amazed or in wonderment as to "How and Why." And yes, it will be the same old questions, "What happened to your leg?" Or, "Does it hurt?"

Therefore, hold on to your faith that sometimes things happen for a reason. And just maybe you are here to help someone else along the journey of life.

Do you believe in ghosts? The answer is yes, I do! But not the traditional Casper the Friendly Ghost or the more scary ghouls that are illustrated in the movie *Ghostbusters*. The ghost I am talking about is a real pain, sometimes called ghost pains, but the medical industry term is phantom limb pain, or PLP. Ghost pains, or PLP, refer to the ongoing sensations that are coming from the part of the limb that was separated from the body or that is no longer there. In my case, that part of my leg below the knee, which is no longer there. I can be just sitting in my recliner or lying in bed, and I can feel the pain in the amputated leg. I sometimes feel like I can wiggle my toes or roll my ankle at times. I personally do not know if it is a psychological issue or the body longing for the missing limb.

Here is a funny thing that happened to me at least once. It was a few weeks after the amputation of the lower left leg. I was in bed and told my mind I was going to the bathroom, so without thinking, I spun around and tried to stand up without the prosthetic leg. And I barely caught myself on the adjoining dresser, or it would have been for me the old saying that I am so fond of: "Down goes Fraser!" I had to laugh to keep from crying. All I can say is, "Yet by the Grace of God goeth I" (Corinthians 15:10).

When a young couple plans to have a baby, they sit up all night thinking about all the supplies and accessories that they will need to make their precious bundle of joy comfortable. Yes, having a healthy baby is a blessing; in the biblical days, a woman was considered truly blessed by God to give birth. (See Genesis 1:28.)

God blessed Adam and Eve and said to be fruitful and increase in number, fill, and subdue the earth. With all that being said, parents must acquire the baby bed or crib, their bottles, diapers, car seat, stroller, baby bags, food, carriers, etc. Therefore, after my surgeries began, guess what? I needed a whole at-home lifestyle readjustment. Just like the baby, I required many items to make my lifestyle at home more comfortable.

Here are the adjustments: If your vehicle's make or model is low to the ground, it can be your primary transportation source for the patient back and forth to all medical appointments. Next, careful thought must be used if you have steps leading to and from your home. A fall is an extreme setback to the at-home rehabilitation efforts or plans. Next, chairs that you plan to sit in must be amenable or conducive to sitting for extended periods, and also, getting up out of a chair can be burdensome.

So, just like a baby, using the potty is a process of trial and error. Making my way to the restroom and using the facilities was an extreme challenge. The first step in the process was to get a portable bedside chair, which could be used anywhere in the house. Yes, it required my wife to do a lot of emptying and cleaning. After several weeks of this procedure, I progressed to using the family toilet but not without needed adjustments. The original unit was too low to the ground. Therefore, we had to order a chair to fit and sit over and above the original toilet. Thank goodness it has a cushioned seat and handrails for easy access.

Lastly, was the adjustment we needed for the bathtub and shower, which was the installation of the shower bench. Early on, I always had bandages on my left foot or leg. I could only shower with my left leg outside of the bathtub. Eventually, we installed handrails around the bathtub, and

I could maneuver to the shower independently. The bathtub is a perilous place for any person with disabilities, man or woman; one missed step or slip can kill you. Yet, But God! We like to say positive thinking and faith in God is our Key! But please add positive pre-planning.

The Ironic Joy Of Thriving Through Devastation

As I mentioned earlier, Rhonda and I started our own distributorship of pain relief products. The ironic part of this new venture is that it was the pain related to the sugar experience that opened doors and pathways to our decision to start delving into selling others pain relief products! Even though there are hundreds of pain relief companies on the Internet, Facebook, radio, and television, amazingly, I discovered that there is a huge market seeking relief from chronic pain.

Several of our customers have tried traditional pain relief products that were on the market! But no actual relief! We gave out several free samples of our products: massage cream, bath salts, lotions, and sprays. The results from the sampling phase were outstanding. Our products outperformed many of the pain relief products that they had previously used. Also, Rhonda and I were users of our products as well! When pain occurred or flared up in our bodies, our products at Nature's Best arthritis and muscle pain relief were always first choice. See our product line and testimonials.

Thriving post-surgery is an ongoing battle. Life itself is man's daily fight against seen and unseen obstacles! First thing in the morning, as you prepare for your daily routines, everything is going to be simply fine, as many theological preachers, pastors, and encouragement specialists will quote. For many, just surviving the day is the goal, one day at a time! Everyone has their own metrics as to what thriving post-devastation means. It could be enjoying family, grandkids, church life, business, sports, travel, public testimonials, etc.

As for me, in the war against "THE SUGAR," it is a return to near normalcy, returning to do most of the things I used to do, but at a different, slower pace. Even without going through a devastating incident like amputation of a lower limb, as co-occupants of our society, we all share the same illness called "THE HUMAN CONDITION," and also the aging process has a big part in our diminished skills and talents.

In closing, be determined to stay in the game of life. I hope my experiences will help you in your life's ENDEAVORS!

ALTHOUGH BLESSED TO BE THRIVING, "I AM STILL A CONTINUAL WORK IN PROGRESS."

Overtime

BISHOP VICTOR SHARPE
ST. JOHN THE GREAT BAPTIST CHURCH
DETROIT, MI

When life's battles against the Sugar have come to a crescendo peak, and when life is hanging in the balance scales of time between life and death—also known as the win-or-lose moments in sports—along comes a heavenly blessing. You hear that still, small voice that says, "Hang on, Help is on the way, and God is not through with you yet!"

Pressing Forward After The Storm

I do not know about you, but in the vernacular language of many people, it is said that "Life Be Lifing." I know this is grammatically incorrect, but that is how people are saying it. I have heard this phrase used repeatedly while talking and listening to people.

I was intrigued by it and decided to research the etymology of the phrase. It is not found in a traditional dictionary, so I resorted to a non-traditional source. So let me paraphrase what I discovered. A lot of the days of our lives are not ordinary; many are full of difficult tasks and very strange occurrences that do not normally happen. Storms of life will come. Life is going to happen no matter what, and the days are going to go on no matter what. So then, all we can do is handle how we're reacting and navigating through obstacles and storms that have come our way. The storms of life are going to take their course.

Life is going to be life, which brings storms, but we get solace in the Word of God, which says, "And we know that all things work together for the good to them that love God, to them who are called according to His purpose" (Romans 8:28).

The Bible oftentimes uses storms as metaphors. From the calming of the tempest to the lessons learned in the raging storm, these stories offer us insight into resilience and faith. While Jesus and His disciples were on the ship, a great storm came, and the Bible says in Mark 4:39, "And he arose, and rebuked the wind, and said unto the sea, Peace, be still. And the wind ceased, and there was a great calm." This gives us the assurance of divine presence during turbulent times and reminds us to trust Jesus the Christ.

Storms have purpose; suffering has benefits. Here are some keys to pressing forward during and after the storm:
1. Know that storms must be embraced as instructors of our faith—trials are weights that make us stronger if we allow them. Turbulence is a teacher.
2. Decide that there are lessons that only storms can teach us—storms always work something in us: patience, experience, hope, and they either break us or build us. It is our choice.
3. 3. Know when to find shelter—your storms are seasonal, so it is necessary to watch the forecasts. See how things are starting out and where you are moving.
4. 4. Set your mind on soaring instead of sulking in sorrows. The characteristics of the eagle remind us that we must learn to navigate through storms.

- Exceptional eyesight—focus is your superpower; do not lose it.
- Resilience—eagles can soar at great heights with strength and resilience.
- Perseverance—keep it moving; that's when power comes.
- Independence—they hang with eagles. Instead of sitting and waiting for the storm to pass, eagles use

the storm to their advantage by going higher, soaring above it—they soar above the storm.

Finally, after the storm, look back and see how the Lord brought you through. We will realize that if it had not been for the Lord, where would we be? Many of our testimonies will be like Apostle Paul; we made it through the storm on broken pieces. Praise God!

Bishop Victor E. Sharpe, Jr. Servant
St. John the Great Cathedral
Detroit, Michigan

Post Amputation Issues

1. The Prosthetic Leg Fitting Procedure
2. Pre-and Post-Surgery Footwear Adjustments
3. Pre-Surgery Vein Procedures
4. Post-Amputation Surgery Allergies
5. Covid Infection Avoidance
6. The Benefits of Being Designated as Disabled

Prosthetic Leg Fitting Procedures

After my leg amputation, I used the advice of my Greek doctor about preparing the remaining stump part of my leg. I had to go through several steps to get the stump ready to receive the prosthetic leg, such as repeatedly beating the stump with a rolled magazine to toughen it up. First, the doctor would wrap my leg with wet-to-dry wrappings or coatings to form a leg cast. Similar to what doctors do when you have a broken leg or arm. I had never had a broken bone or limb. Therefore, I did not know what to expect. I thought the initial wrap would be a part of my prosthetic leg, and I would walk out of the doctor's office the same day with a new leg. Silly me, a novice to medical or post-surgery procedures.

I had to wait about fifteen minutes or so for the cast to dry, and to my amazement, it was rock hard; the technician quickly removed it, and it was a replica of my stump. They explained to me this was the foundation scale that would be used to create the prosthetic leg. So, I asked, "When will it be ready? Will it be 2–3 days?" The technician said that based on how my insurance company approves the procedure, the plan would determine whether it would take up to five or six weeks. I was semi-floored because I had high expectations of walking as soon as possible. I am highly hyper, even though I do not show a hyperactive outside personality. But inside, I am a raging bull of hyperactivity.

Once again, I left the doctor's office in my wheelchair, severely depressed. Yes, I was knocked down in my emotions but not defeated in the battle. Patience is a well-learned virtue. The ability to wait or endure something without getting upset is a positive trait or virtue.

Pre-And Post Surgery Footwear Adjustments

Pre-surgery: My infected foot swelled from a shoe size thirteen to a new size fifteen. I had to buy two different shoe sizes for several years: the left foot was size fifteen, and the right foot was size thirteen.

Post-surgery: After several surgeries, a strange thing happened with my shoe sizes. Even though I was wearing a size thirteen pre-surgery, my right foot, now the weight-bearing skeletal foot, was and is a size fifteen. Therefore, you can say I grew into a size fifteen. The company that collaborated with me on my prosthetic leg proposed making the prosthetic foot a size fifteen. This would allow me to balance my walking, running, jogging, etc. I would have a quality sense of balance with the same shoe sizes. I can say the commonly known expression "a pair of shoes, not two pairs." The other caveat about the same shoe size on both feet is that it helps with my balance; it helps me navigate uneven surfaces, going up hills and coming down hills.

Pre-Surgery Procedures

Leg vein blockage or rotor-rooter vein procedure.

I often developed cramps in the back of both of my legs after just running. Usually, I could run all day and drink lots of water or rehydration fluids like Gatorade, and the cramps would go away. All of a sudden, I would be walking with no real extension, my legs would become stiff, and I would have to sit until the pain subsided. I was already taking blood thinners to regulate blood flow. Something was wrong, so I asked my general practitioner what was causing the frequent leg cramps. First, he recommended going to a heart doctor for testing. I said to myself, "But why would there be a need for me to see a heart doctor?" I was not having chest pains; I thought that was what they checked the heart for-—signs of heart attack and strokes.

But, when I arrived, they informed me that the first series of tests was checking for blood pressure stress on the blood and that my heart was circulating blood throughout the body from head to toe regularly. Wow, was I surprised at the stress procedures they did! They put monitors on both legs and both forearms, and then they cranked up the pressure, and my heart started to race faster and faster. I thought I was going to pass out! I was forewarned that this was a normal reaction from these tests. I said, "Lord, let me get out of here ASAP!" But I had to wait until the injection of whatever heart-racing medication that they gave wore off.

Alarming, at first, they said it looked like I had a vein blockage in my heart muscles. So, I consulted with the heart specialist, who recommended stents to be placed in my heart to relieve the pressure and allow more accessible blood flow through the heart. This should alleviate the cramping in my legs. So, that stent operation procedure was set in place. The day I showed up and went under anesthesia, something unusual happened. I woke up and asked, "How did the stent procedure go?" The heart specialist said it turned out that I did not need stents. It was only a calcium buildup. I left his office scratching my semi-bald head, wondering what was next. He recommended that I see a vein specialist or an intravenous radiologist. I asked, "What would they do that you did not do?"

So, weeks turned into months, and one fateful morning, I woke up with blisters on all my toes. Then, I knew it was time to see the intravenous radiologist, or jokingly the roto-rooter doctor. My wife researched and found a good one and set the appointment; he performed similar pressure tests on both my legs and forearms. He determined that I had a vein blockage in my legs. I said, "Are you going to put stents in my legs?" He informed me that it would be a more invasive procedure. Boy, did that announcement scare me. He explained what my wife calls the rotor-rooter procedure. This is where they insert a small device starting at your waist that goes down through the groin area and down to your toes. Yes, I could feel this device, although I was under a mild anesthetic. Thus, I was awake during the entire procedure, and, funny thing, the nursing assistants would ask me every few minutes if I needed more pain medication, and I would always say yes.

The situation reminded me of an airplane trip that I took several years ago on a seagoing airplane. Let me explain that while boarding the aircraft, the flight attendant would ask each passenger how much they weighed and how many bags they checked for the trip. As the curious George, I asked, "What does it matter how much a person weighs?" She kindly explained that the bags' weight plus each passenger's weight helped the pilot determine how much fuel to add to the tank. I asked myself, "Why don't they just fill it up in case of trouble?" The story's moral is for the attending nurses during my procedure to give me the highest dose of the pain medication just in case trouble arises. In other words, fill it up!

So, I walked out of the procedure sore throughout my lower body. They told me not to lift anything or stress my body out in any way for a couple of days; you see, the roto-rooter helped stop my cramps temporarily. The procedure was clearing all the veins and arteries, removing any blockage of blood flow.

Post-Amputation Surgery Food Allergies

Yes, soon after my lower leg amputation, I developed strange food allergies. I used to love eating watermelon and cantaloupes, but now I throw up whenever I try to consume these two fruits. I also have a negative reaction when I eat too much shrimp, shellfish, or crab legs. I start to swell in my ankles when I eat these in abundance. I go on a roller coaster ride with weight loss and gain.

Yes, with my condition, I have to take a daily juggernaut of medication; most of these medications work together and have a good working relationship with each other. I consume pills for blood pressure, diabetes injections five times a day, appetite suppressants, water pills to help my swelling, stool softeners, and, of course, Tylenol for pain relief. My wife is tasked with ensuring these medications are taken correctly. Yes, at times, I felt like the proverbial Five Million Dollar Man—this movie casts a severely injured man who was rebuilt through a secret government agency. Water retention or fluid buildup was a significant issue for my joints. This contributed to my roller coaster effect of weight gain and loss. You do not have to starve yourself.

Covid Infection Avoidance

Let me speak a little about my journey during the COVID years. I was always conscious that the infection could kill me. I was an extremely faithful member of our church during the height of the Covid years of exposure. I admit that I feared attending church regularly on Sundays for two years. But I kept the faith and kept up with our minimal church activities via the internet broadcast. Even with life-threatening effects like COVID-19, the work of the church must continue. Yes, we were only contributing financially with our weekly tithes and offerings. As time passed and the disease's effects decreased, we eventually went back to worship. Apostle Paul wrote that it was good to do good and help people with disabilities, infirmities, sickness, depression, and the poor, as long as the work does not cause you to become one of them. (See 1 Corinthians 9:15.)

He also spoke about giving up your self-imposed rights for those weak in their faith. Remember God's words: whoever is kind to the poor and the infirmed lends to the Lord, and He will reward them for what they have done. Therefore, even if misfortune or adversity comes your way, be kind to everyone because no one caused your malady. The theology of life's adventures is "that God wills it or allows it to happen to you." Just ask Job. And God can deliver you out of it.

Benefits Of Being Designated As Disabled

Yes, life has its difficulties. Adversity is never really pre-planned; sometimes, it just happens. But if you are willing to accept God's blessings in your life, you must also accept God's vengeance and wrath. You cannot take the good things and leave the bad. Humorously, here are a few benefits of being disabled:

1. You get the best parking spots at stores, restaurants, and civic events.
2. You ride in motorized carts in big box stores, airports, and more.
3. You get front-row seats at the movies and concerts.
4. You get to go first on the airplane.
5. You always sit in the non-smoking areas.

But these benefits are not free; you must be willing to give up an arm or a leg! Finally, my wife says that as hard as I try to stay in good shape, I have developed a "granddad body."

Contributors

Dentistry—Ronald T. Blanchette, DDS
1. DIABETIC VISION AND EYE CARE
2. General Practitioner—Dana J. Wright, MD
3. Anesthesiology—Marilyn L. Treadwell, CRNA
4. Spiritual Empowerment During Challenging Times—

Dr. Frank E. Ray, Sr.
1. Spiritual Preparedness for Enduring Times—

Reverend Albert Bry, Jr.
1. The Power of Consistent Prayer During Perilous Times—
2. Bishop Kevin Treadwell
3. Modern Day Miracles—Reverend Martin Treadwell

Endocrinology

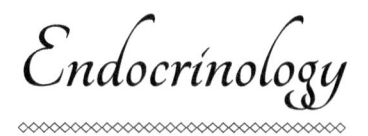

What is Type 1 diabetes?

Type 1 diabetes is an autoimmune disease that occurs when the cells in the immune system attack insulin-producing cells in the pancreas called beta cells.

This is a branch of biology and medicine dealing with the endocrine system. It is a disease, and its specific secretions are known as hormones. It is also concerned with the integration of developmental events, proliferation and psychological or behavioral activities of metabolism, growth and development, tissue function, sleep, digestion, respiration, excretion, mood, stress, and lactation movement. Hormones cause reproduction and sensory perception. All are factors involved with diabetes. The doctor who manages diabetic care is known as an endocrinologist.

An endocrinologist provides diagnoses and care for health issues rooted in the endocrine system, such as evaluating diabetes, bone loss, and a range of hormonal issues, including issues from the pituitary and adrenal, thyroid glands, as well as reproductive organs.[2]

High blood glucose is also known as "hyperglycemia." The glucose level is considered high when it is 160 mg/

dL above your individual blood glucose target. Be sure to ask your healthcare provider what (s)he thinks is a safe target for your individual glucose level both before and after meals.

People with Type I Diabetes have extremely high blood sugar levels (250 mg/dL) upon diagnosis. For a person with diabetes, hyperglycemia is usually considered to be a blood glucose level greater than 180 mg/dL one to two hours after eating. But this can vary depending on what your target blood sugar goals are.

A healthy (normal) fasting blood glucose level for someone without diabetes is 70 to 99 mg/dL (3.9 to 5.5 mmol/L).

Dental Hygiene

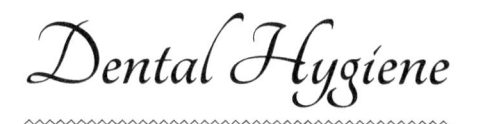

The SUGAR affects so many areas of your body—even your mouth. Diabetes can affect your teeth, gums, tongue and all the soft and hard tissue in your mouth. Keeping a healthy mouth and managing your blood glucose level goes hand and hand.

People with diabetes should make sure they have regular dental checkups. Getting your teeth cleaned regularly at the dentist, brushing at least twice a day, and flossing at least once a day can help keep your mouth healthy and keep inflammation and infection in your mouth under control.

Diabetics can have oral health problems: gum disease (periodontal disease), dry mouth, thrush, slow healing after any gum surgery, bad breath, and tooth loss. If you smoke—STOP. It is not good for your oral health, and it is not good for your overall health.

Having good oral health is a big part of keeping your diabetes under control.

Diabetic Vision And Eye Care

If you have diabetes, you already know that your body can not process or store sugar properly. When your blood sugar is elevated, it can cause damage to the blood vessels in your eyes. The medical term for this condition is diabetic retinopathy. The longer someone has diabetes, the more likely they are to have retinopathy or simply damage to the retina from the disease.

Generally, diabetics do not develop diabetic retinopathy until they have had the disease for at least ten years. As soon as you have been diagnosed with diabetes, you need to have an eye examination at least once per year. It is essential to know you cannot diagnose diabetic retinopathy by looking in the mirror, since your eyes will usually look and feel normal despite the presence of a potentially blinding condition. Only a complete and thorough retinal examination and screening will help detect if you have issues. By the time you notice vision changes from the effects of diabetes, your eyes may already be irreparably damaged. So, routine eye examinations are highly important. In most cases, your eye or vision specialist can detect signs of diabetes even before you notice any visual symptoms. Early detection and treatment can prevent vision loss.

Early detection of any malady or disease is the number one "tenet" of the medical industry. It is always better to do preventive care versus aftercare.

Anesthesiology

Diabetes and Anesthesia

Anesthesia providers should perform a thorough history and physical prior to administering anesthesia to diabetic patients. It is estimated that one quarter of diabetic patients are unaware they are diabetic. Another study revealed that 7.4 percent of patients undergoing surgery were unaware of their diabetes.

Pertinent information would include, and is not restricted, to what type: Type 1 versus Type II

Medication regimen: oral antihyperglycemics, non-insulin injectables, insulin, sodium-glucose cotransporter-2 inhibitors (SGLT-2), and glucagon-like peptide-1 receptor agonists (GLP-1) Hemoglobin A1C result.

Glucose control: are you monitoring at home; at what glucose level do you experience hypo/hyperglycemia?

Related complications: neuropathy, kidney disease, retinopathy, cardiovascular disease.

Anesthesia complications: difficult intubation due to arthritic complications.

Many hospitals and ambulatory facilities schedule diabetic patients as the first cases of the day or as early as possible in order to prevent prolonged fasting periods. It is pertinent for patients to follow the preoperative instructions, such as:

NPO guidelines: no food after midnight. This is important as diabetes can sometimes cause delayed gastric emptying, which increases the risk of aspiration.

Medications: you may need to decrease insulin doses by 20–25 percent. Some medications should be held the night before, such as metformin. Other medications, such as GLP-1, should be held for a week and the SGLT-2 inhibitors for seventy-two hours. Failure to follow preoperative guidelines can result in cancellation or delay of the procedure, which is inconvenient to the patient and family.

Out-of-range lab values can also result in same-day cancellations. Hyperglycemia, or high glucose, can result in the same-day cancellation of procedures. Cancellation on non-emergency procedures should be considered for A1C levels of 7–9 or glucose 300-500 mg/dl. An elevated A1C indicates undiagnosed diabetes or poorly controlled diabetes, which increases the risk of delayed wound healing, infections and an increase in morbidity and mortality. It may be in the best interest of the patient to reschedule the procedure for a few months and seek the advice of an endocrinologist to achieve better diabetic control.

Hypoglycemia, or low blood sugar, carries its own set of risks. Some of the risks include neurological damage, cognitive decline, and other serious issues. Some of the symptoms of hypoglycemia are difficult to detect under anesthesia whether it is general versus sedation. This is why it is imperative that patients share the level of which they experience symptoms. Anesthesia providers continue to monitor blood glucose during the anesthetic and post-anesthesia recovery period. Each patient is unique, and the more information given about the diabetic management helps the care team, as the patient is the expert of their care. Although many of the questions seem redundant and a bit frustrating, patient participation and a thorough history and physical are necessary to provide the best care.

Marilyn L. Treadwell

Certified Registered Nurse Anesthetist (CRNA)

Masters of Science in Nursing (MSN)

Doctorate of Nursing Practice (DN)

Home Health Care Perspective

Diabetes and home health…*in my little practice nurse opinion.*

Home health for diabetics can be helpful in situations where there is a need for therapy, education, wound care, and/or medication management.

Home health offers a bit more of a holistic view of a patient's life. Health care providers can assess aspects of a patient's physical, mental, social, emotional, environmental, and economic state as well as provide in-home medical care and observation. Nurses, doctors, CNAs, and social workers work together to identify the need for referrals for community resources and social services.

The goal of the home health team is to reduce visits to the ER and reduce hospital stays—in other words, it is a resource to help keep people healthy at HOME.

Care /Case Managers offered by the health insurance plan or Medicare Advantage plan can help with patient advocacy, medication costs, transportation issues, and even help with community resources such as housing and food. Weekly or monthly visits or calls by nurses are done for care and monitoring.

Things a nurse thinks are important:

Rule #1 – Keep all your doctor's appointments.

Rule #2 – Always be brutally honest. The BEST advocate for anyone is themselves when it comes to changes, concerns, or just questions.

Rule # 3 - Find providers that agree with your mind, body, AND spirit. Everyone is not compatible. Compatibility and trust are important. Please do not stay with a provider that is not good at listening or explaining.

Diabetic Education

All individuals diagnosed with diabetes and their caregivers should attend diabetic education classes so that an individual can learn more about diet and lifestyle modifications needed to live a healthy and active life. It is important that an individual knows how to read nutrition labels and identify areas where they may be consuming excess sugar in hidden places, like drinks such as juice and colas.

Ask PCP for diabetic education classes and report back the status of the wound. Since the risk of infection is so high, regular wound care is needed and extended antibiotic therapy may be needed by oral therapy or by

IV therapy.

Since some wounds need an extended amount of time to heal, a PICC or midline may be placed at a medical facility so that long term antibiotic therapy can be administered at home. These are IV lines that stay in place for the duration of the medication therapy. The home health nurse will monitor the patient for any signs of infection or side effects and report the patient's progress to the doctor. Home health nurses are responsible for the dressing changes associated with these types of IV lines since there is a high chance of infection. Some medications can be administered by the patient and the family, while some medications can only be administered by the nurse.

Blood Pressure

Uncontrolled diabetes + uncontrolled hypertension = kidney damage. High blood pressure is just as serious as diabetes. It is so important to follow both diabetic and heart healthy diets. Keeping a home BP cuff is vital. Whenever there is a dizzy spell or an unusual headache, check BP! Keep a record of readings and share it with your PCP.

Hydration

Stay hydrated. Kidneys are important. So is beautiful skin while we age. If your doctor has you on fluid restrictions, FOLLOW IT. Water is water. Tea is not water alone anymore. Cola is not water alone anymore. Coffee is not water alone anymore.

Medications

Medication reminders and pill boxes are a helpful tool for everyone.

It is best to have all your medications filled with one pharmacy. A person could be receiving a brand name medication at one pharmacy and a generic from another, thinking it is a different medication when they are taking double the dose that the doctor ordered for them. This can be EXTREMELY dangerous and even fatal, as some medications increase the chances of getting dizzy and falling.

DO NOT SKIP MEDICATIONS!!! If you are unsure about a medication, contact your doctor's office and ask questions. Be open and honest about concerns and any noticed side effects or changes since starting or stopping any medications. If medications are too costly, there are programs through the medication manufacturers that can help with costs. Insurance plans often have diabetic testing supplies at low or no cost. Ask nurses at your doctor's office about these programs as well.

Candice R. Hathaway
Licensed Practical Nurse (LPN)
Nashville, TN

Pictorial Journey

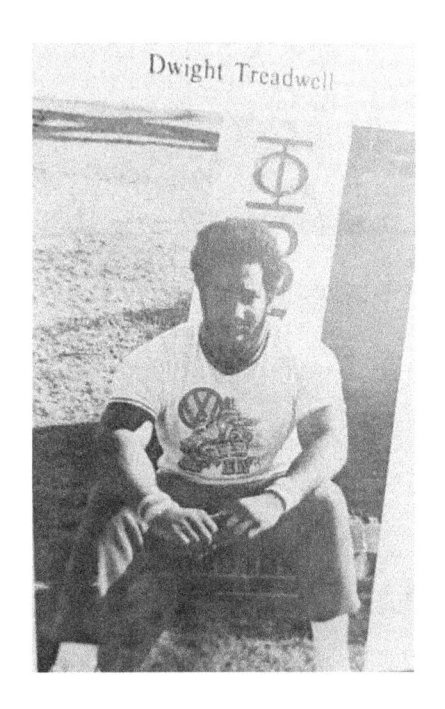

Knoxville College, 1973

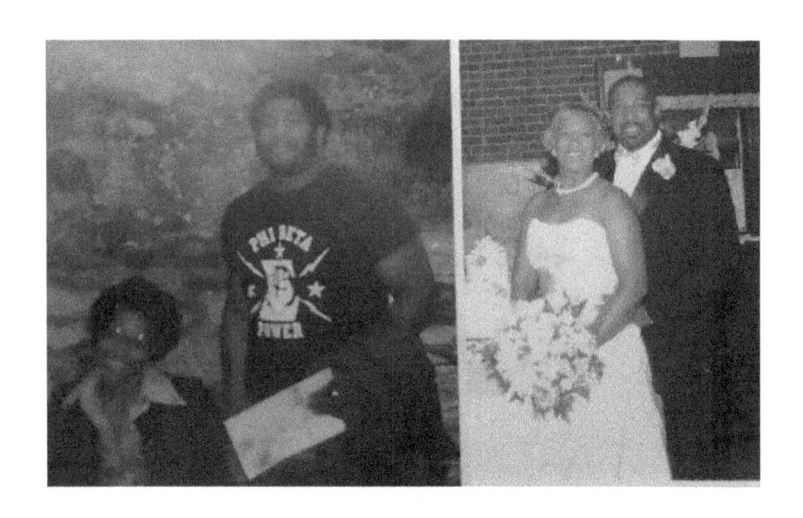

Rhonda and Dwight, 1977 and 2007

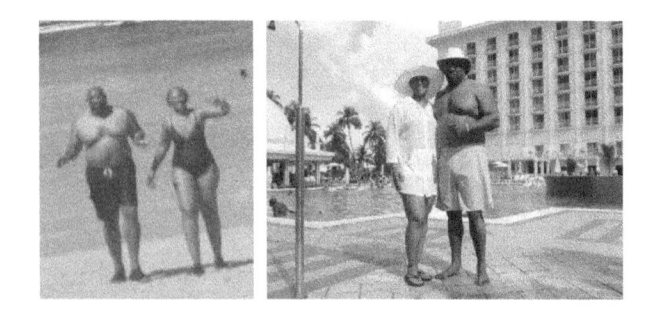

Vacationing, 2009 and 2010

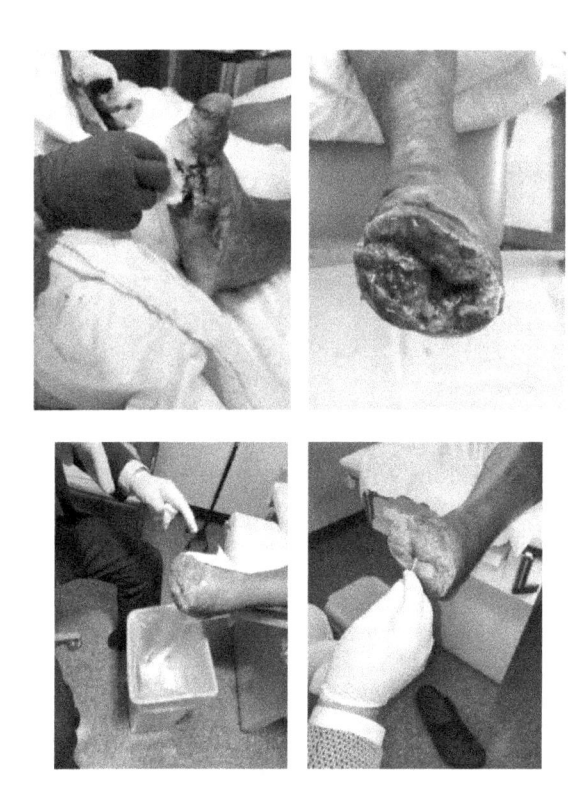

Four-and-a-half-year journey of saving the foot and leg.

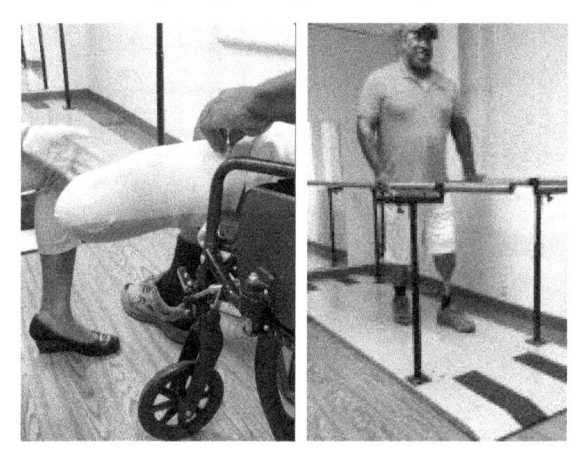

Getting fitted with the first prosthetic leg and learning how to walk.

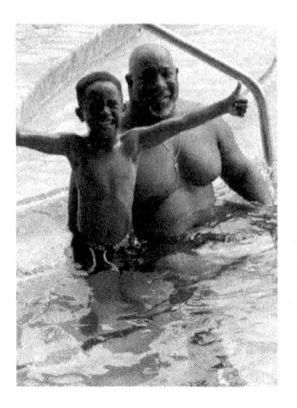

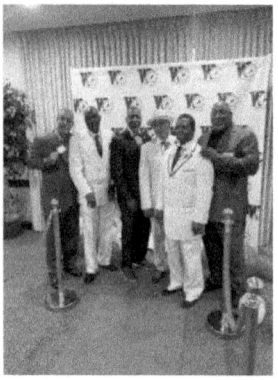

Swimming with Grandson and attending 50th High School Reunion

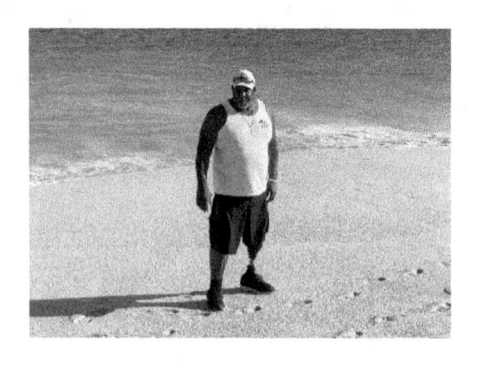

2024

Testimonials

I do not have diabetes myself, but many of my cousins do! Diabetes seemed to have skipped me. The book is a great read and a great tool for diabetics to read! The Sugar is an amazing journey of your life's ups and downs.

Melvin S.

Overcoming and Thriving from the Devastating Effects of "The Sugar," aka Diabetes by Dwight Treadwell shares a deeply personal account of the author's experience managing and living with diabetes. Treadwell approaches the subject from a lived perspective, detailing both his physical struggles and the emotional impact of the disease. The book aims to offer readers not only insights into the challenges of managing diabetes but also inspiration to push through obstacles with resilience and hope.

Treadwell highlights the complications and lifestyle adjustments diabetes often demands. His story is one of transformation, with insights into how he coped with symptoms and found strategies to improve his quality of life. This book appeals to those directly affected by diabetes and their families, as it offers guidance, encouragement, and an understanding of the disease's reality from someone who has endured it firsthand.

If you're interested in an honest look at the day-to-day experiences of managing diabetes, Treadwell's narrative provides a blend of hope and practical advice. It's available through various online retailers and offers a window into the author's journey toward resilience and self-care.

G. Carter

If you're interested in an honest look at the day-to-day experiences of managing diabetes, Treadwell's narrative provides a blend of hope and practical advice. It's available through various online retailers and offers a window into the author's journey toward resilience and self-care.

David G

At the close of another day, we must acknowledge that there are several individuals who can master unknown mysteries, who can delve into the complexity of the atom, who tower high in academic excellence, and those who can speak many languages fluently. But no one can tell your story like you can!

The Bible teaches us that to achieve, you must believe in the Power of Faith through Prayer. The spoken word has great power. But the written word shall live on through eternity.

Thank you for "The Sugar" book. You have had quite a challenge for sure. I have read it through twice and fully understand what you have gone through. I can relate, with having diabetes myself and having a sister succumb to this disease with an amputation and loss of her sight.

Thanks for sharing your story! I'm sure this will bring encouragement to someone going through this experience.

D. Northcut

Dwight, your book has been very informative and very inspiring to me. Having just lost a son to diabetes, it truly touched my inner soul. You never realize how this disease can affect you until you or someone you know has been affected by it. I am borderline and must keep a close check on myself. God bless you for this book.

G. Taylor

Congratulations, my friend! I'm thrilled for you; your story will inspire anyone else suffering through the process.

L. Watson

I just finished your book. I enjoyed it. Your mother and wife are a blessing, and you have a wonderful support group.

Incorporating Rhonda's story as a caregiver significantly enhanced your book. Her perspective on turning a job loss into a positive outcome is compelling and inspiring.

I understand how neuropathy and pain tolerance became a war by itself, and not getting hooked on that morphine had to be a challenge.

B. Ingram

Man, I'm not a reader by nature, but today I sat and read your awesome book on "The Sugar" from cover to cover. Tread, your story is a tribute to your drive & determination, Rhonda's love for you and God's will. Thanks so much for prompting me to read it. It's an easy read & your humor had me giggling in the midst of learning of your struggles to prevail. I'm encouraged by your message and pray God continues to cover you & Rhonda in this thing we call LIFE.

K. Lee

Conclusion

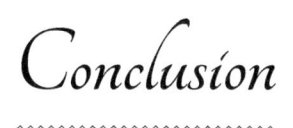

Even though the Bible is seen as one book with many interesting stories, it is a book of many well-timed, interwoven mini-stories injected into major themes. The mini-stories are not usually major events by themselves! For instance, when Jesus was approached by Jairus, the leader of the Pharisees, about his daughter who was sick almost unto death! This unusual encounter between the two opposing leaders on this day was the major story!

But, as Jesus was on His way to Jairus' home, He ran into a woman who had been sick for twelve years with an incurable blood disease! Jesus stopped in the middle of a crowd of followers to ask the question: "Who Touched Me?"

This mini-story only serves to set the tone of God! He cares about the rich and the poor! So, God is never too busy to hear your prayers!

Jesus' message to the leader of the Pharisees and the unknown woman regarding the issue of blood was the same! "Only Believe."

The unknown woman was not a major story! She didn't even have a name! Nobody even knew where she came from! She was never mentioned again in the Bible! She was just a part of the Pharisee leader's story!

So, in conclusion, you might look back over your life and ask, "Am I the major story in this life? Or am I a mini-story in someone else's life?" Whatever the case may be, whether you are a major player in a storyline or just a minor player, you are injected into the major story. Yes, the mini-stories are usually not connected directly to the major story! They are just miraculously placed pawns and injections! Yes, in this Christian walk of life, we are just glad to be used as pawns for God to help someone else realize how He uses people to bless other people, in their journey to serve and to understand God's purpose for their lives!

"The Power of Faith Through Prayer"

Endnotes

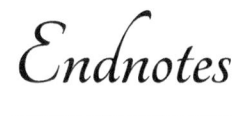

1 Blackaby, Richard. 2015. "Experiencing God Day by Day (Devotional) - PDF Free Download." Epdf.pub. EPDF.PUB. 2015. http://www.epdf.pub/experiencing-god-day-by-day-devotionalfbee3968130ff8ff5b968b-819344c92d54004.html.

2 Wikipedia Contributors. 2019. "Endocrinology." Wikipedia. Wikimedia Foundation. March 21, 2019. https://en.wikipedia.org/wiki/Endocrinology.

3 "Perioperative Management of the Diabetic Patient: Overview, Physiology of Glucose Metabolism, General Preoperative Assessment." 2019. Medscape.com. November 9, 2019. https://emedicine.medscape.com/article/284451-overview.

Bibliography

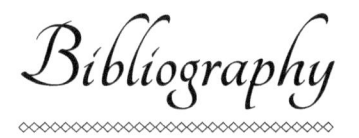

CDC. 2020. "Centers for Disease Control and Prevention." Centers for Disease Control and

Prevention. February 13, 2020. http://www.cdc.gov.

Cleveland Clinic. 2023. "Diabetes." Cleveland Clinic. February 17, 2023.

https://my.clevelandclinic.org/health/diseases/7104-diabetes.

"Joslin Diabetes Center." 2024. Joslin.org. 2024. https://joslin.org/.

Loh-Trivedi, Mira. 2024. Review of *Perioperative Management of the Diabetic Patient*.

Medscape. July 24, 2024. https://emedicine.medscape.com/article/284451-overview.

"Medscape: Diabetes & Endocrinology." n.d. Www.medscape.com.

https://www.medscape.com/diabetes-endocrinology.

"National Center for Biotechnology Information." 2019. Nih.gov. 2019.

http://www.ncbi.nlm.nih.gov.

"Sacramento Dentist — Ronald T. Blanchette, DDS — Sacramento, CA." 2024. Ronald T.

Blanchette, DDS. December 29, 2024. https://sacramentocadental.com/.

"Total Eye Care, P.A." 2021. Eyecare. June 29, 2021. https://www.totaleyecarememphis.com/.